HANDBOOK OF
PEDIATRIC MOCK CODES

HANDBOOK OF
PEDIATRIC MOCK CODES

Editors

MARK G. ROBACK, M.D.

Assistant Professor, Department of Pediatrics
University of Colorado School of Medicine;
Department of Emergency Medicine
The Children's Hospital
Denver, Colorado

STEPHEN J. TEACH, M.D., M.P.H., F.A.A.P.

Assistant Professor of Pediatrics and Emergency Medicine
George Washington University School of Medicine;
Department of Emergency Medicine
Children's National Medical Center
Washington, D.C.

LEWIS R. FIRST, M.D., F.A.A.P.

Professor and Chairman, Department of Pediatrics
University of Vermont College of Medicine
Burlington, Vermont

GARY R. FLEISHER, M.D., F.A.A.P., F.A.C.E.P.

Professor of Pediatrics, Harvard Medical School;
Chief, Emergency Medicine, Children's Hospital
Boston, Massachusetts

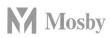 Mosby

St. Louis Baltimore Boston Carlsbad Chicago Minneapolis New York Philadelphia Portland
London Milan Sydney Tokyo Toronto

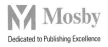

Mosby
Dedicated to Publishing Excellence

A Times Mirror
Company

Editor: Kathryn H. Falk
Project Manager: Patricia Tannian
Book Design Manager: Gail Morey Hudson
Manufacturing Manager: Dave Graybill
Senior Composition Specialist: Peggy Hill
Cover Design: Teresa Breckwoldt

Printed in the United States of America
Composition by Mosby Electronic Production
Lithography by Top Graphics
Printing/binding by R.R. Donnelley & Sons Company

Mosby–Year Book, Inc.
11830 Westline Industrial Drive
St. Louis, Missouri 63146

Library of Congress Cataloging in Publication Data
Handbook of pediatric mock codes / editors, Mark G. Roback . . . [et al.].
          p.   cm.
     Includes bibliographical references and index.
     ISBN 1-55664-452-3 (softbound)
     1. CPR (First aid) for children. 2. CPR (First aid) for children—Study and teaching. I.
Roback, Mark G.
     [DNLM: 1. Resuscitation—in infancy and childhood. 2. Resuscitation—education.
   WS 100 H232 1998]
   RJ370.H37 1998
   618.92'1025-dc21
   DNLM/DLC
   for Library of Congress   97-37730
                                                                               CIP

98 99 00 01 02 / 9 8 7 6 5 4 3 2 1

Contributors

ANDREW M. ATZ, M.D.
Assistant in Cardiology
Children's Hospital;
Instructor in Pediatrics
Harvard Medical School,
Boston, Massachusetts

RICHARD BACHUR, M.D.
The Children's Medical Group
Poughkeepsie, New York

KATHLENE BASSETT, M.D.
Assistant Clinical Professor,
Department of Pediatrics
University of Colorado School of Medicine;
Section of Emergency Medicine
The Children's Hospital
Denver, Colorado

PAUL BOURESSA, M.D.
PeaceHealth Medical Group
Eugene, Oregon

DAVID BROUSSEAU, M.D.
Fellow, Emergency Department
Hasbro Children's Hospital
Brown University School of Medicine
Providence, Rhode Island

LYDIA CIARALLO, M.D.
Emergency Department
Hasbro Children's Hospital;
Assistant Professor of Pediatrics
Brown University School of Medicine
Providence, Rhode Island

KATHRYN D. CLARK, M.D.
Assistant Professor
Department of Pediatrics
University of Colorado School of Medicine;
Section of Emergency Medicine
The Children's Hospital
Denver, Colorado

FRANCES CRAIG, M.D.
Clinical Instructor in Pediatrics
University of Utah School of Medicine;
Fellow, Pediatric Emergency Medicine
Primary Children's Medical Center
Salt Lake City, Utah

CARLOS A. DELGADO, M.D.
Associate Fellowship Director
Division of Pediatric Emergency Medicine
Assistant Professor of Pediatrics
Emory University School of Medicine
Atlanta, Georgia

ALLAN DOCTOR, M.D.
Fellow in Critical Care
Children's Hospital
Harvard Medical School
Boston, Massachusetts

GLENN FARIES, M.D.
Assistant Clinical Professor
Department of Pediatrics
University of Colorado School of Medicine;
Section of Emergency Medicine
The Children's Hospital
Denver, Colorado

LEWIS R. FIRST, M.D.
Professor and Chairman
Department of Pediatrics
University of Vermont College of Medicine
Burlington, Vermont

GARY R. FLEISHER, M.D.
Associate Professor of Pediatrics
Harvard Medical School;
Chief, Emergency Medicine
Children's Hospital
Boston, Massachusetts

KAREN GRUSKIN, M.D.
Division of Emergency Medicine
Children's Hospital
Harvard Medical School
Boston, Massachusetts

ERICA LIEBELT, M.D.
Director, Pediatric Emergency Services
Penn State Geisinger Health System
Danville, Pennsylvania

CHARLES MACIAS, M.D.
Assistant Clinical Professor
Department of Pediatrics
Baylor College of Medicine;
Section of Emergency Medicine
Texas Children's Hospital
Houston, Texas

HOLLY PERRY, M.D.
Assistant Professor of Pediatrics
University of Cincinnati College of Medicine;
Division of Emergency Medicine
Children's Hospital Medical Center
Cincinnati, Ohio

KRISTINE RITTICHIER, M.D.
Fellow, Section of Emergency Medicine
The Children's Hospital
University of Colorado School of Medicine
Denver, Colorado

MARK G. ROBACK, M.D.
Assistant Professor
Department of Pediatrics
University of Colorado School of Medicine;
Section of Emergency Medicine
The Children's Hospital
Denver, Colorado

RICHARD A. SALADINO, M.D.
Assistant Professor in Pediatrics,
Harvard Medical School;
Division of Emergency Medicine
Children's Hospital
Boston, Massachusetts

ANNE M. STACK, M.D.
Instructor of Pediatrics
Harvard Medical School;
Assistant in Medicine
Children's Hospital
Boston, Massachusetts

STEPHEN J. TEACH, M.D., M.P.H.
Assistant Professor of Pediatrics and Emergency
Medicine
George Washington University School of Medicine;
Department of Emergency Medicine
Children's National Medical Center
Washington, D.C.

GUY L. UPSHAW, M.D.
Assistant Clinical Professor
Department of Pediatrics
University of Colorado School of Medicine;
Section of Emergency Medicine
The Children's Hospital
Denver, Colorado

JOE WATHEN, M.D.
Fellow, Section of Emergency Medicine
The Children's Hospital
University of Colorado School of Medicine
Denver, Colorado

DEBRA L. WEINER, M.D., Ph.D.
Instructor of Pediatrics
Harvard Medical School;
Assistant in Medicine
Children's Hospital
Boston, Massachusetts

To
**all those who care for ill and injured children
and to our families
for their love and support.
À Hélène et Emma, avec tout mon amour.**

Preface

Society has witnessed a dramatic fall in the death rate for children during the past century. This epidemiological miracle has had a profound impact on our thinking as parents and on our performance as pediatricians and emergency physicians.

It's a shock when a child dies, especially when the death occurs suddenly or unexpectedly. Physicians accept the eventuality of death for their oldest patients, and even family members are unlikely to question nature's wisdom when relatives finally succumb to long, drawn-out illnesses. But it's different with infants and children. Advances in health care have led parents as well as physicians to expect that every youth will survive through adolescence. Evidence of this transformation in thinking appears in our daily newspapers: a single fatality of a child from meningococcemia in a small community reverberates to the four corners of a state within a day.

Residents and nurses in training seldom witness the death of a child, except neonates and children with do-not-resuscitate orders. Sudden infant death syndrome, the number one cause of mortality in infants after they leave the newborn nursery, has declined dramatically since the simple but elusive connection with sleeping position was discovered. In the protection of children beyond the age of one year, when trauma takes over as the chief culprit in pediatric deaths, society has made dramatic strides as well. The use of passenger restraints, bicycle helmets, and safer packaging for hazardous medications has contributed to a marked decline in fatalities. Added to these advances, the movement (perhaps ill-founded) of many resuscitations in the prehospital arena has led to a generation of trainees with minimal exposure to the resuscitation of children.

Yet physicians are likely to be called upon to resuscitate a child on one or more occasions in their careers. And during their training, the anxiety that exists around the possibility of this occurrence is evident. Residents want and need competence in pediatric resuscitation.

The dichotomy between the wants and needs of residents, medical students, and nurses on the one hand and a declining opportunity to gain adequate experience on the other confronts educators at many institutions. Faced with this problem, Children's Hospital in Boston began the "Mock Code" Program under the direction of Dr. Paul Wise in the early 1980s. Dr. Lewis First inherited the program 15 years ago and combined his medical knowledge and theatrical talent to further develop this program to assist participants in acquiring the psychomotor and attitudinal, as well as cognitive, skills of pediatric resuscitation. With each new class of residents the scenarios for the mock codes became more elaborate. Advancing technologies, such as arrhythmia generators, have added a new dimension to the process.

The development of a fellowship in pediatric emergency medicine (PEM) provided a seemingly endless supply of enthusiastic practitioners of mock codes. Eventually Mark Roback and Stephen Teach as fellows and new PEM attending physicians in Denver and Buffalo took on the challenge of translating an oral tradition into written words. From these origins arose the present volume, the *Handbook of Pediatric Mock Codes*.

While most readers are probably familiar with the concept of mock codes and some may even have had firsthand experience with them, users will find this text unique. Its aim is to transform the current practice of teaching resuscitation from an informal process of questionable value to a science with defined methods and clear-cut goals. The introduction lays down the ground rules for using the material. The core of the text is 37 scenarios covering the breadth of pediatric resuscitation. Although the more frequent events, such as trauma and respiratory arrest, are emphasized, less common pediatric problems, from electrocution to complications of pregnancy, are also included.

If one thinks of a mock code as a type of play, the special qualities of this book become apparent. Producers need interesting characters, creative dialogue, and detailed stage directions to put on successful shows. Similarly, educators require realistic case scenarios, interventions leading to appropriate responses, and instructions for the orchestration of various simulations to stage an effective mock code. In this text each of the scenarios includes a case presentation, a description of likely suggestions for treatment and outcomes, a discussion of possible complications, and a review of the specific lessons to be learned. The depth, quality, and logical formatting of the material provide the substrate for a superb educational program in resuscitation that has been refined through 15 years of continuous use. We hope that the *Handbook of Pediatric Mock Codes* will eventually lead to standardized teaching of CPR for children and, in addition, will provide a tool for evaluating competency across institutions.

Mark G. Roback, M.D.
Stephen J. Teach, M.D.
Lewis R. First, M.D.
Gary R. Fleisher, M.D.

Acknowledgments

I wish to acknowledge the pediatric life support courses on which this text is based; Dr. Al Tsai, who introduced me to pediatric emergency medicine; and Dr. Joe Stenzel, who first showed me the educational value of the mock code exercise.

A special thank you to Dr. Gary Fleisher and Dr. Lewis First, whose mentoring has played a major role in my development as a physician.

I would also like to thank F. Keith Battan, M.D., David Brousseau, M.D., and Carol Okada, M.D., for their thoughtful reviews of this work.

Mark G. Roback, M.D.

Contents

How to Use This Handbook

The purpose of the mock code exercise is to reinforce management of the ABCs (airway, breathing, and circulation) of resuscitation as learned in basic and advanced life support courses. This handbook describes how a successful mock code program may be initiated. The goal of such a program is to make participants proficient in management of the ABCs and to decrease their anxiety about pediatric resuscitation through creative simulation and repetition. Mock code programs should be flexible and can include pediatric, surgical, emergency, and family medicine residents; nurses; medical students; paramedics; emergency medical technicians; respiratory therapists; and pharmacists. These participants gain experience resuscitating pediatric "patients" in 37 situations, or mock code scenarios. The book gives step-by-step directions for conducting mock codes in a wide variety of patient care settings.

Chapter 1, Guidelines for Conducting the Mock Code, provides the nuts and bolts for the book. This chapter explains in detail how to run mock codes. It defines the roles of the participants and lists the materials required to make the mock codes as realistic as possible. Most important, this chapter suggests ways to modify the mock code exercise to fit the specific needs of the participants and institution. The mock code exercise may be used effectively in a wide variety of settings, from the academic pediatric medical center to the general pediatrics or family medicine clinic.

Chapter 2, Common Interventions and Complications, provides examples of common interventions, complications, or progressions of pediatric disease. Before conducting a mock code the educator may refer to this section for ideas to be used in any given scenario. Advanced management techniques are also discussed.

Chapter 3, Mock Code Scenarios, offers 37 life-threatening situations for resuscitation practice. The list encompasses a wide range of childhood illnesses and injuries that practitioners may have to address at some time. Each scenario provides complete information for performing the exercise, including detailed progression options, expected responses, complications, and outcomes. Objectives are discussed at the end of each scenario with additional comments on selected topics. References are provided for further study.

The mock code scenarios are designed to facilitate flexibility. It is vital that those who use this book be able to modify the scenarios to meet the needs of their facility. Each scenario offers options applicable to the experience level of the participating mock code teams. Certain scenarios offer several variations, the focus of which is left up to the mock code director. All the mock code scenarios may be changed appreciably by subtly altering the history, physical examination, or progression of disease.

The scenarios are divided into eight categories. The first three, Airway, Breathing, and Circulation, encompass fundamental and common pediatric emergencies. These are presented in a basic, straightforward manner for the beginner. Options are offered to challenge more experienced participants. For example, in the Airway Foreign Body scenario, recognition of airway obstruction and removal of the foreign body suffice in the most simple case. Options range from hypoxic insult leading to full arrest requiring intubation and resuscitation, for advanced beginners, to airway obstruction requiring a surgical airway, for the more expert participants.

The remaining five categories of mock code scenarios address emergencies with specific presenting complaints. Neurologic scenarios deal with such problems as altered mental status, seizure, and headache. Cardiac emergency scenarios focus on patients with arrhythmias and cyanosis. The trauma, environmental, and pregnancy-related emergency scenarios consider specific situations, injuries, and disease entities.

Following the scenarios section is **Chapter 4, Initial Approaches,** which summarizes for quick reference the approaches to and algorithms for basic problems encountered in the scenarios. This book focuses on recognition and management of emergency situations. We have listed several excellent references for in-depth study of specific topics.

Our goal is to present a handbook that may be used by anyone involved in the care of seriously ill or injured children. All that is required to make the scenarios work in any given situation is a good idea of the experience level of the participants and a little imagination.

1 Guidelines for Conducting the Mock Code

OBJECTIVES

As discussed in "How to Use This Handbook," the objective of the mock code is to furnish clinicians with experience in caring for seriously ill or injured pediatric patients. Participants receive practice in situations that require immediate attention to the ABCs (airway, breathing, and circulation) of pediatric resuscitation. A transition from basic to advanced life support techniques is inherent in every mock code.

In addition, each mock code scenario has three or four distinct objectives. Individual mock codes stress specific aspects of resuscitation, such as airway obstruction, respiratory distress, and shock. Initial assessment and management of the ABCs are required at the onset of every mock code. This may be followed by a progression of disease or injury that may enlist any of the complications in Chapter 2.

MOCK CODE TEAM PARTICIPANTS—ROLES AND RESPONSIBILITIES

Not all patient care facilities have the luxury of fully staffed critical care areas for a complete, formal code team (Box 1-1). Many variations of the model described below exist, and an institution can easily incorporate whatever resources are available to make up its own mock code team. For example, many of the "physician" positions may be filled by nurses, respiratory therapists, physician assistants, paramedics, or emergency medical technicians, depending on the setting. Similarly, residents or medical students may take on roles typically filled by nurses. We have successfully conducted mock codes with one nurse and one doctor participating. All members of the code team are important, and their performances will be reviewed.

BOX 1-1

MOCK CODE PARTICIPANTS

Code team
- Team leader
- Nursing staff
- Physicians
- Ancillary staff

Mock code director

Reviewer(s)

We have found it helpful to give a formal lecture at various times of the year (to account for rotating staff) to orient members of the code team to their individual responsibilities and expectations regarding performance in the mock code. We stress that this is an educational experience, acknowledge the fact they will feel stressed, and generally make every effort to set a collegial tone to the exercise.

Team Leader

- Identifies self as the person responsible for directing members of the code team (assigns roles to physicians and nurses).
- Asks for consulting services (general surgery, neurosurgery, orthopedics, radiology, etc.) as indicated.
- Is responsible for crowd and noise control.
- Ensures utilization of "universal precautions."

Airway Physician

- Is responsible for control of the airway with rigorous attention to protection of the cervical spine.
- Provides assisted ventilation and intubates when necessary.
- Assesses mental status and pupillary response.
- Assesses the head for signs of trauma.

Physician on Patient's Right

- Provides right-sided IV access and blood draw for laboratory studies.
- Performs right-sided procedures (e.g., chest tube, NG tube, Foley catheter).
- Performs cardiac compressions when indicated.

Physician on Patient's Left

- Performs the primary survey, a 60-second physical examination.
- Provides left-sided IV access and blood draw for laboratory studies.
- Performs left-sided procedures (chest tube).
- Performs the secondary survey, a more detailed examination including rectal examination and examination of the patient's back.

Float Physician

- Obtains the initial history.
- Communicates the history to the team leader.
- Is available for cardiac compression relief.
- Acts as a liaison between the code team and parents or family members.

Medication Nurse

- Calculates the weight of the patient in kilograms.
- Anticipates and draws up medications quickly and accurately, including the first round of resuscitation medications, which are labeled by hand.

- Communicates directly with the team leader *only* regarding administration of drugs.
- *Orally* states the name and dosage of each drug before handing it over to the person administering it.
- Prepares continuous-infusion drugs and sets up arterial lines.

Bedside Nurse

- Is responsible for the primary survey.
- Is responsible for vital signs, monitors, oxygen, and suction.
- Assists with procedures.
- Administers IV medications.

Documenting Nurse

- Documents dosage and time of all drugs given and informs the team leader.
- Keeps track of length of the arrest and the patient's response to therapy.
- Documents and labels all laboratory specimens.
- Documents vital signs every 5 minutes.
- Is responsible for fully completing the arrest flow sheet.

Circulating Nurse

- Assists with management of airway and cervical spine immobilization.
- Assists with IV access, IV infusions, and arterial line setup.
- Pages consulting services when asked by the team leader.

Nursing Assistants

- Report to the documenting nurse for direction.
- Send specimens to the laboratory and obtain blood products, equipment, or drugs.

Mock Code Director and Reviewers

The mock code director (MCD) interacts with the code team in such a way as to focus attention on the ABCs and the objectives of the specific scenario offered in the mock code exercise. Further duties of the MCD and the reviewer's role are described later in the chapter.

EQUIPMENT

The equipment used for the mock code need not be elaborate and should be recycled. The presence of the physical objects to be used is essential, but some supplies can be displayed without being opened. For example, it is sufficient for a code team member to describe how an IO needle is placed while holding an unopened needle. However, newer mannequins can be used to demonstrate actual procedures such as endotracheal intubation and IO placement, and in this instance use of actual materials adds greatly to the experience. Care must be exercised when actual needles are used.

Similarly, resuscitation drugs that might be required should be available but the medication nurse need only describe the volume of a given concentration of drug to be drawn up without actually doing it. Having the drugs on hand so that participants may view the size and shape of vials as well as volumes and concentrations is essential.

BOX 1-2

EQUIPMENT LIST FOR PEDIATRIC RESUSCITATION

Mannequins (pediatric sizes)
Monitors: ECG and oximeter, blood pressure cuff
Backboard and hard cervical spine collars
Airway equipment
- Oxygen source with tubing
- Suction with catheters
- Bag-valve-mask apparatus
- Oral airway, nasal trumpet
- Laryngoscopes, endotracheal tubes, stylets

Vascular access equipment
- IVs of various sizes
- IO needles
- Central venous catheter line (CVL) kits
- IV fluid bags

Resuscitation drugs
Rhythm generator (see Appendix E, ECG Rhythms, p. 218)
Defibrillator with pediatric attachments
Orthopedic splints
MAST trousers
End-tidal CO_2 monitor

BOX 1-3

ADDITIONAL EQUIPMENT REQUIRED FOR NEONATAL RESUSCITATION

Radiant warmer or warming lights, warm blankets or towels
Cardiorespiratory monitor, temperature probe
Suction catheter (5 Fr) and suction source with gauge
Anesthesia bag with manometer or self-inflating bag with pop-off valve
Face masks (preterm and term)
Oral airways (000-01)
Laryngoscope (Miller 0 and 1 blades)
Endotracheal tube (2.5-4.0) with stylet
Stethoscope (newborn size appropriate)
Cord clamps and scissors

The practice of opening and using resuscitation equipment may be made cost effective by saving opened equipment in a mock code supply box. The box is brought out before each mock code, and its contents are distributed appropriately for reuse. At institutions where the exercise occurs frequently a mock code crash cart may be set up so all equipment and drugs necessary for resuscitation are readily available.

Note: Care must be taken to ensure that the mock code supply box or mock code crash cart is never inadvertently opened and materials used in a real resuscitation.

Equipment and medications useful in the mock code exercises are listed in Boxes 1-2 to 1-4. It is not essential that all the listed equipment and medications be available to perform a successful mock code. The MCD should use what is available and stress the ABCs.

BOX 1-4

MEDICATIONS

Oxygen
Normal saline or Ringer's lactate solution
Dextrose solutions
Epinephrine 1:10,000 and 1:1000 concentrations
Atropine
Paralytics and sedatives (see Rapid Sequence Intubation, p. 10)

BOX 1-5

TIME SCHEDULES FOR MOCK CODE

60-Minute Mock Code	Elapsed Time in Minutes
Setup	Before exercise
Introduction	0-5
Scenario	5-20
Review/questions	20-40
Demonstration of skills	40-60

30-Minute Mock Code	Elapsed Time in Minutes
Setup	Before exercise
Scenario	0-15
Review/questions	15-30

SCENARIOS

The mock code scenarios are designed to be realistic and practical. If the participants believe the events may actually happen to them someday, they will have much more invested in the process. The scenarios should be kept simple in the beginning. The participants will indicate by their responses what their level of experience is and how complicated any scenario may become.

A strict 15-minute time limit is enforced for the actual scenario. The rest of the time is devoted to setup, review, and questions. The entire exercise may be designed to last either 30 or 60 minutes. Demonstrations of skills (intubation, vascular access, etc.) may take place at the end as time permits or after the allotted mock code time (Box 1-5).

The MCD is responsible for arriving well before the scheduled start of the exercise to prepare the mannequin and set up the resuscitation equipment. Diligence in preparation is important to a successful program.

The MCD begins each exercise by summoning the code team to the patient (mannequin) area. A brief introduction may be given to stress to participants the need to address the mannequin as if it were a real patient. This means that if a participant wants to know what the lungs sound like, he or she should already have auscultated the chest using a stethoscope. It should be emphasized that all information required may be obtained from the MCD. The MCD acts as the parents (during the history), gives physical findings when asked, and describes the patient's progression and response to interventions made by the code team.

A useful option is to alternate between physicians and nursing staff as to who is allowed to address the "patient" first. After initial assessment the starting group is required to call the other for assistance. This emphasizes the need for a complete code team and stresses to all members the value of collaborative care.

It is the duty of the MCD to orchestrate the movements of the mock code. The MCD begins the mock code scenario by delivering a brief initial history. As the team begins the initial assessment and management, the MCD gives additional information only when asked by the team or team leader. Requiring the team to elicit information (history, physical examination) and to describe procedures (indications, landmarks, equipment) is a major objective of all mock code exercises.

When giving information the MCD should use specific numbers and historical data, for example, "The heart rate is 190 bpm" rather than "The patient is tachycardic." The use of actual numbers gives the scenario an essence of reality and allows the MCD to change the vital signs as the scenario unfolds. Team members take the exercise more seriously when specific information is offered.

The MCD must maintain a balance between giving information not elicited by the team and allowing them to stray too far afield. The MCD may nudge the team back on course by adding a timely bit of information or may emphasize a point by allowing the mock code to progress to full cardiopulmonary arrest.

ENDING THE MOCK CODE EXERCISE AND PATIENT DISPOSITION

When the patient's condition has been stabilized, the MCD must bring the exercise to a formal end. One effective method of closure is to ask the team leader, "Now what?" At the point when the code team members recognize that patient disposition is in order, the mock code scenario has reached an acceptable end.

Alternatively, the MCD may say, "OK, let's stop." The team leader is then questioned regarding patient disposition. Besides serving as a form of closure, this allows further insight into the team leader's assessment of the situation. For example, if the team leader believes a floor bed is adequate for a patient who obviously needs the OR, something is awry.

Disposition options typically include the hospital ward, ICU, CT scanner, or OR. The morgue is not an option. Mock codes should never end in the death of the patient, since mannequin deaths greatly detract from the learning experience. The participants become so focused on the act of dying that the objectives of the mock code exercise become secondary. Trainees should emerge from the process feeling empowered, not defeated.

If the MCD wants the code team to experience "death of a patient," as in an unsalvageable case of sudden infant death syndrome (SIDS), the exercise should have no other objectives. The

ABCs of resuscitation are lost on participants when the outcome is death. Giving participants experience in dealing with the death of a patient is a worthwhile objective but is beyond the scope of this book.

REVIEW

The effectiveness of the mock code experience may be enhanced by having an observer, preferably someone of superior training and experience, watch the mock code proceedings and assess the performances of the participants. This reviewer then discusses the responses of physicians and nursing staff in the mock code. The review, focusing on teamwork and covering the objectives of the given scenario, should last no more than 15 to 20 minutes.

If no additional person is available to serve as the reviewer, the MCD may fill this role. When the MCD is also required to be the reviewer, it is important that he or she be very familiar with the given scenario. Intimate knowledge of the scenario and its objectives should facilitate the difficult duty of performing both roles simultaneously.

Ideally the mock code is a positive learning experience for all participants. When giving feedback the reviewer should initially stress the positive aspects of each mock code exercise. He or she should emphasize what has been done correctly before launching into the areas where improvement is needed.

The mock code checklist (see Appendix A, p. 210) may be used as a review guide. It emphasizes the ABCs and the primary and secondary survey. The mock code checklist specifies important information that should be gathered and tools that may be needed in any code situation. The reviewer may find it convenient to refer to the checklist and to record notes on it during the mock code.

During the review the code team should receive *no more than three main issues* on which to focus their attention for future improvement. The reviewer should stick to the basics, stressing the ABCs and objectives and not getting hung up on style points or minutiae.

It is important to allow the code team members opportunity to ask questions regarding the mock code and their performance. This may take place during or after the reviews. Reviews should be given in an educational manner that fosters questions and discussion. The 15- to 20-minute time limit must be kept in mind.

Giving feedback effectively is an art. Every effort should be undertaken to make the mock code exercise a learning experience. The relative inexperience of many of the participants necessitates conducting reviews in an upbeat fashion. We encourage anyone conducting mock codes to investigate further resources for methods of giving feedback. Two excellent references are provided at the end of the chapter.

CLOSING STATEMENTS

In closing, the MCD summarizes the scenario, the team's response, and the reviews. He or she should again stress the objectives of the scenario, repeat the diagnosis, and briefly discuss the initial management and progression. The MCD is responsible for ending the event on a positive note. Procedures encountered may be further explained and demonstrated after the MCD's closing statements.

KEEPING TRACK

A well-organized longitudinal pediatric mock code program should have a quality assurance and improvement component. Records may be kept of the date, location, scenario used, participants, and their performance in each mock code. Notes may be taken on particular strengths and weaknesses of each exercise, as well as participants' responses. By referring to these notes, coordinators can gain insights into how future mock code exercises may be run better and participants may be helped to improve their resuscitation skills.

REFERENCES

Ende J: Feedback in clinical medical education, *JAMA* 250:777-781, 1983.

Weinholtz D, Edwards JC: Providing feedback. In *Teaching during rounds*, Baltimore, 1992, Johns Hopkins University Press, pp 85-93.

2 Common Interventions and Complications

The following is a list of basic interventions and complications that may arise in any resuscitation situation. They may be used in any of the mock code scenarios and are presented to reinforce the ABCs of pediatric resuscitation (Box 2-1).

BOX 2-1

ABCs OF RESUSCITATION

A—**Airway**, with attention to control of the cervical spine
B—**Breathing**
C—**Circulation**
D—**Disability** (brief neurologic assessment)
E—**Exposure** ("If you are sick enough to be resuscitated, you need to be naked.")

A—AIRWAY

With attention to control of the cervical spine when trauma is suspected.

Assessment

Is the patient able to speak or cry?
Look: For respiratory distress, choking, or cyanosis that may indicate airway obstruction.
Feel: For movement of air from mouth and nose.
Listen: For air movement over the airway (throat) and quality of breath sounds (stridor).
     As the team addresses the airway, equipment to be assembled includes:
- Oxygen, face mask, nonrebreather, bag-valve-mask as indicated.
- Suction equipment with appropriately sized catheters.
- Airway management devices (see below).

Interventions

I. Management of airway obstruction. Avoid anatomic obstruction (hypopharyngeal tissue block) by:
- Midline position of the head.
- "Sniffing" position (slight extension of neck, contraindicated in trauma).
- Controlling the tongue: Chin lift, jaw thrust.

- Removing secretions and vomitus: Suction, log-roll the patient with in-line immobilization when indicated to protect the cervical spine (see III. Cervical Spine Immobilization, p. 11).
- Oral airway and nasal trumpet: When the patient has good respiratory effort but has mechanical obstruction despite the above maneuvers.

Complications
- Oxygen and suction tubing not connected to wall.
- Oxygen flow inadequate.
- Suction catheter too small.

II. Endotracheal intubation

Indications. Cardiopulmonary arrest, apnea, respiratory insufficiency, actual or potential airway obstruction, respiratory depression, severe burns, severe multiple trauma, severe head injury, increased intracranial pressure (ICP), depressed mental status, and loss of normal protective airway reflexes.

- Laryngoscopy and intubation may result in bradycardia, pain, ICP elevation, increased risk of gastric regurgitation and aspiration, and hypoxia.
- Assemble materials required for intubation: 100% oxygen, suction, bag-valve-mask, laryngoscope (with functioning light) and endotracheal tube (ETT) of proper size. ETT size estimation: **(age + 16) divided by 4** (see Appendix C, p. 214).

Rapid sequence intubation (RSI). Performed for patients with full (or presumed full) stomachs to achieve a fully relaxed state for ease of intubation and fewer adverse effects. Proceed in the following manner:

1. Preoxygenation: 100% inspired oxygen for 2 to 5 minutes.
2. Vagal stimulation blocker (also reduces oral secretions): Typically used empirically in children less than 5 years or with associated bradycardia. Patients less than 5 years of age receiving the paralytic succinylcholine may experience significant bradycardia, making the use of atropine mandatory before administration of succinylcholine.
   Atropine 0.02 mg/kg IV
3. Ensure a good mask seal over the mouth and nose. Be prepared to perform bag-valve-mask ventilation if the initial intubation attempt fails.
4. Apply cricoid pressure (Sellick maneuver) to occlude the esophagus (antiemesis technique) without compressing the airway or moving the cervical spine. Cricoid pressure should be used in any patient receiving positive-pressure ventilation (includes bag-valve-mask).
5. Drugs of RSI include:
   Sedative to induce unconsciousness options.
   Midazolam 0.1 to 0.3 mg/kg IV.
   Thiopental 2 to 5 mg/kg IV.
   Ketamine 1 to 2 mg/kg IV.
   Muscle relaxant options.
   Succinylcholine 1 to 2 mg/kg IV.
   Vecuronium 0.1 to 0.2 mg/kg IV.
   Pancuronium 0.1 to 0.15 mg/kg IV.
   Rocuronium 0.6 to 1 mg/kg IV.

6. When ICP elevation is a concern, lidocaine may be used.
   Lidocaine 1 mg/kg IV.
7. **Fentanyl** 2-5 µg/kg IV is often used in the RSI as an adjunct to sedation, although its primary effect is analgesia.
8. Attempt intubation when full airway muscle relaxation is achieved.
9. Confirm ETT placement:
   Look: Watch the ETT go through the cords! Look for condensation in the ETT and symmetric chest rise.
   Listen: For symmetric breath sounds and over the abdomen.
   Observe: The patient's response, heart rate, skin color.
   Monitors: Pulse oximeter, end-tidal CO_2.
   Confirm: CXR, ABG.
10. Use NG/OG tube to evacuate stomach (cricoid pressure is maintained until placement of tube is confirmed by auscultation).

Note: The drugs used in any given RSI vary depending on specific patient problem, experience of physicians administering the drugs, and individual and institutional preferences. In the following scenarios the drugs listed reflect the authors' preferences for the given situation. Other drugs may be substituted safely in most cases. Distinct contraindications are discussed.

Complications

- Emesis (may occur during assisted ventilation or just before intubation): Requires proper use of suction with maintenance of cervical spine immobilization where appropriate (log-rolling patient).
- Failure of laryngoscope light.
- Decreased or absent breath sounds on the left, suggesting a right mainstem intubation.
- Esophageal intubation.
- Extubation if the ETT is not properly handled and taped.

III. Cervical spine immobilization. Proper cervical spine immobilization includes:

- Hard cervical collar. (Soft cervical collars offer *no* protection to an unstable cervical spine.)
- Full spine board.
- Taping or strapping of head, trunk, and pelvis to a hard board.

Complications

- Improper in-line immobilization before obtaining cervical spine control.
- Improper cervical spine collar size or type used.
- Head not secured in place (towel rolls or sandbags placed on either side of head must be taped or strapped to the backboard).

IV. Endotracheal tube medications. LEAN—*L*idocaine, *E*pinephrine, *A*tropine, *N*aloxone.

V. Cricothyrotomy

Indications. Airway obstruction resulting in increasing desaturation, cyanosis, bradycardia, and impending cardiorespiratory failure when conventional methods of securing the airway (endotracheal intubation) are unsuccessful. Percutaneous needle or catheter cricothyrotomy results in effective oxygenation but poor ventilation.

1. Place a 14- to 16-gauge Angiocath through the cricothyroid membrane. Connect the Angiocath to the oxygen tubing using the hub from a 3.0 ETT for transtracheal ventilation.
2. Connect to 100% oxygen at 50 psi (15 L/min).
3. Deliver intermittent bursts at a rate of approximately 20 per minute. Each burst lasts about 1 second on (inspiration) followed by 2 seconds off (exhalation).
4. Use a jet ventilator if available.

B—BREATHING
Assessment

Look: For symmetric chest rise, use of accessory muscles, and skin color.

Listen: Auscultate breath sounds for adequate air movement, symmetry, quality of breath sounds, and presence of extra sounds such as stridor, crackles, or wheezes.

Monitors: The pulse oximeter is good for *oxygenation* (Po_2) only and tells nothing about ventilation (Pco_2). The end-tidal CO_2 monitor is used for the noninvasive assessment of ventilation.

Interventions

I. Bag ventilation

- Positive-pressure ventilation is delivered via a self-inflating or an anesthesia-type **Ambu** bag. (The anesthesia type requires an oxygen source for inflation.) Bag ventilation must always be performed *with 100% oxygen.*
- Bag-valve-mask (BVM) ventilation requires proper head positioning and a good seal on the face with a properly sized face mask and an Ambu bag of appropriate volume.
- Bagging an intubated patient requires a properly sized (appropriate volume) Ambu bag and a good connection with the ETT.
- Effectiveness of bagging must be assessed by observing chest excursion, auscultating breath sounds, and monitoring vital signs and pulse oximeter readings.
- All patients receiving positive-pressure ventilation are at risk for:
    1. Aspiration of stomach contents; cricoid pressure must be applied.
    2. Abdominal distention from air, which may compromise ventilation; an NG or OG tube is required.

Complications

- Face mask that is wrong size for patient; poor seal results in ineffective oxygenation and ventilation.
- Ambu bag that is the wrong size, resulting in underventilation or overventilation.
- Overzealous bagging or use of an oversized Ambu bag, leading to pneumothorax.
- Vomiting, leading to aspiration if no cricoid pressure is used.
- Abdominal distention resulting from bagging, necessitating an NG tube.
- Air leak from a small ETT, resulting in ineffective ventilation.

II. Thoracentesis

Indications. Thoracentesis is a lifesaving intervention used in cases of suspected tension pneumothorax. As a temporizing measure done before chest tube placement, thoracentesis may also be performed to remove fluid (a chest tube is typically more effective).

- Use an anterior approach for air: sterile prep, second intercostal space in the midclavicular line, 22- to 18-gauge catheter.
- Use a posterior approach for fluid: midaxillary line, fourth or fifth intercostal space.
- Always introduce the needle superior to the rib to avoid the intercostal neurovascular bundle, which runs deep to the thinner, inferior aspect of the rib.
- Have a T-connector, three-way stopcock, and 60 ml syringe setup readily available.

Complications. Pneumothorax or hemothorax, pulmonary contusion, hepatic or splenic trauma.

III. Thoracostomy tube

Indications. Traumatic pneumothorax, hemothorax, or hemopneumothorax.
- Discuss landmarks: just anterior to the midaxillary line at nipple level, over the rib.
- Appropriate tube size: see Appendix C, p. 214.
- Appropriate setup of chest tube suction.
- Never place a chest tube through a penetrating wound.

Complications. Pneumothorax or hemothorax, pulmonary contusion, hepatic or splenic trauma, damage to the long thoracic nerve or mammary tissue.

C—CIRCULATION
Assessment

Look: The patient's color (pink, mottled, ashen, pale, or cyanotic) gives important information about perfusion. Capillary refill time is less than 2 seconds centrally in patients with adequate perfusion.

Feel: Assess the quality of pulses. Palpate the brachial artery in infants. Palpate the femoral or carotid pulses in toddlers and older children.

Monitor: CR (cardiorespiratory) monitor is the most important because tachycardia is an early indicator of shock. Low blood pressure or hypotension is a late finding of shock in pediatric patients.

Interventions

I. Chest compressions

Indications. Asystole or absence of a peripheral pulse; heart rate less than 80 beats/min in a neonate or less than 60 beats/min in an older infant; straight line (asystole) on an ECG monitor *with corresponding loss of pulse and heart rate.*
- Patient resting on a flat, hard surface (backboard).
- Proper positioning and technique (Table 2-1).
- Step (to stand on) if indicated.
- Change of position when fatigued (usually after no more than 5 minutes).

Table 2-1 *Rate and Depth of Chest Compressions*

	Infant	Child	Adult
Compressions (rate/min)	100+	100	80
Depth of compressions (inches)	0.5-1	1-1.5	1.5-2

Complications. Ineffective compressions because of lack of backboard, poor positioning, fatigue, or improper rate or depth of compressions; inadvertent compressions resulting from failure to assess pulses and reliance on ECG monitor that shows asystole (wires disconnected).

II. Venous access

1. Peripheral IV

- The site of choice is the large veins of the antecubital fossae, but in infants and small children the saphenous veins can be used effectively. The external jugular vein is also accessed for resuscitation. Hands and scalp veins may not flow well enough for volume resuscitation but initially may be the only access available.
- Require team members to announce the size of the catheter and the site landmarks before each attempt.
- Require the team to continue to search for an alternative IV access even after the initial line placement is successful.

Complications. Unsuccessful attempt because of an improper size catheter for the patient's age or situation; blown or clotted line because of failure to have an IV line readily available.

2. Intraosseous line

Indications. Emergencies in which intravenous access cannot be obtained or in which time required to obtain intravenous access may significantly alter the chance of survival.

- The Pediatric Advanced Life Support (PALS) course manual recommends that IO lines be placed in patients less than 7 years of age when no other means of venous access are obtainable.
- For practical purposes, peripheral access should be attempted for less than 90 seconds.

Infusion. Fluids (crystalloid or colloid) and most drugs (epinephrine, atropine, sodium bicarbonate, dopamine, diazepam, phenytoin, paralytics, and antibiotics).

Contraindications. Infection at the intended puncture site, fracture of the bone, previous attempt on the same extremity.

Sites

- Proximal tibia: Patients less than 5 or 6 years of age, medial and inferior to the tibial tuberosity with needle pointing in a slightly caudal fashion (away from the growth plate).
- Distal tibia: Preferred site for adults but also good for infants and children; medial surface at the junction of the medial malleolus and the shaft of the tibia.
- Distal femur: When tibia has been attempted or is not available bilaterally, the medial aspect of the distal femur is an acceptable alternative, especially in older patients.

Equipment. A 16- or 18-gauge IO needle. Spinal needles are acceptable but generally too long for effective, rapid fluid infusion.

Complications

- Incorrect landmarks or an improper needle, resulting in an unsuccessful attempt with infusion of fluid into soft tissues.
- Attempt at a second site on the same long bone, leading to major infiltration and unsuccessful infusion of fluid or drugs.
- Fracture.

3. Femoral line

Indications. Used in resuscitation when peripheral venous access attempts are unsuccessful or central access is required.
- Landmarks: NAVL (lateral to medial: *N*erve, *A*rtery, *V*ein, *L*ymph).
- Seldinger (guide wire) technique.

Complications
- Improper landmarks, resulting in arterial puncture or an unsuccessful attempt.
- Arterial puncture, leading to a large hematoma.
- Large catheters in small vessels, leading to compromise of lower extremity circulation.
- Femoral nerve damage.

4. Cutdown

Typically carried out on the saphenous or femoral veins, this procedure, although highly effective for the administration of resuscitation fluids and medications, is generally performed by surgeons and typically reserved for trauma resuscitations. Cutdowns may also be used successfully in medical resuscitations.

5. Umbilical vein cannulation

Indications. Emergency resuscitation and stabilization; administration of fluids, blood, and resuscitation medications to the newborn.

Complications
- Vessel perforation, leading to hemorrhage and inability to perform fluid resuscitation.
- Vasospasm, resulting in unsuccessful arterial line placement.

III. Cardioversion

Indications. Ventricular tachycardia with a pulse, symptomatic supraventricular tachycardia (hypotension, concern that the rhythm may become a malignant one).
- Paddle size: Standard 8 cm adult paddles whenever chest size allows; otherwise 4.5 cm pediatric paddles should be used. Prep paddles or skin electrodes with electrode paste, being careful not to let paste from one site touch the other and form an "electrical bridge" between sites, which could result in ineffective defibrillation and possibly skin burns.
- Sites: Anterior chest wall, on the right side of the sternum inferior to the clavicle and on the left midclavicular line at the level of the xiphoid.
- Energy dose: Synchronous mode, initial dose is 0.5 joules/kg; double dose if unsuccessful. See Chapter 4.

IV. Defibrillation

Indications. Ventricular fibrillation, ventricular tachycardia without a pulse.
- Proper paddle size and placement: Heart between paddles, typically one paddle on the right side of the chest below the clavicle and the other lateral to the left nipple in the anterior axillary line. See III. Cardioversion above.
- Properly charged pack, proper conductive medium, and clearing of area before electrical discharge.
- Energy dose: Asynchronous mode, 2 joules/kg; if unsuccessful, repeat immediately. If still unsuccessful, double the dose (4 joules/kg) and repeat.

- Proper oxygenation, ventilation, and correction of underlying acidosis or hypothermia: These may be required for successful defibrillation. Administration of epinephrine may also improve cardiac perfusion enough to make defibrillation successful. See Chapter 4.

Complications

- Ineffective electricity owing to failure to charge, improper positioning on the chest, or incorrect paddle size.
- Use of improper conduction medium (e.g., alcohol swabs), leading to second-degree burns on the chest.
- Failure to "clear" before voltage discharge, leading to morbidity of a code team member.

ADDITIONAL INTERVENTIONS
1. Diagnostic Peritoneal Lavage

Diagnostic peritoneal lavage (DPL) has been used as an adjunct to the physical examination in an attempt to identify significant intraabdominal injuries. It is not routinely used in children, since a positive result does not necessitate operative management. Splenic and hepatic injuries are frequently managed nonoperatively. One potential indication in children is simultaneous blunt abdominal trauma and head injury in a hemodynamically compromised child. A negative DPL might allow a CT scan of the head to be performed before operative intervention.

The procedure consists of inserting a catheter into the peritoneum and lavaging with sterile saline (15 ml/kg). The lavage fluid is then analyzed for the presence of red and white blood cells, amylase, and alkaline phosphatase.

2. Military Antishock Trousers

Note: The use of military antishock trousers (MAST) in pediatrics is highly controversial. Indications and contraindications for use in adults are listed below.

Indications

- Pelvic fracture splinting and hemostasis.
- Soft tissue hemorrhage tamponade.
- Leg fracture stabilization.
- Circulation stabilization for transport.
- Upper torso perfusion maintenance in the face of inadequate or absent volume replacement.

Contraindications

- Myocardial dysfunction.
- Pulmonary edema.
- Intrathoracic hemorrhage.
- Diaphragmatic rupture.

REFERENCES

American Heart Association, American Academy of Pediatrics: *Textbook of pediatric advanced life support*, 1997.
American Heart Association, American Academy of Pediatrics: *Textbook of pediatric basic life support*, 1992.
Baren JM, Seidel JS: Emergency management of respiratory distress and failure. In Barkin RM: *Pediatric emergency medicine, concepts and clinical practice*, ed 2, St Louis, 1997, Mosby.

Frumkin K, Wright SW: Tube thoracostomy. In Roberts JR, Hedges JR, eds: *Clinical procedures in emergency medicine*, ed 2, Philadelphia, 1991, WB Saunders, pp 128-149.

Ludwig S, Kettrick RG. Resuscitation—pediatric basic and advanced life support. In Fleisher GR, Ludwig S, eds: *Textbook of pediatric emergency medicine*, ed 3, Baltimore, 1993, Williams & Wilkins, pp 1-31.

Mace SE: Cricothyrotomy. In Roberts JR, Hedges JR, eds: *Clinical procedures in emergency medicine*, Philadelphia, 1991, WB Saunders, pp 48-60.

Ross DS: Thoracentesis. In Roberts JR, Hedges JR, eds: *Clinical procedures in emergency medicine*, ed 2, Philadelphia, 1991, WB Saunders, pp 112-128.

Sacchetti AD: Seldinger (guide wire) technique for venous access. In Roberts JR, Hedges JR, eds: *Clinical procedures in emergency medicine*, ed 2, Philadelphia, 1991, WB Saunders, pp 307-314.

Seidel JM: Cardiopulmonary resuscitation. In Barkin RM: *Pediatric emergency medicine: concepts and clinical practice*, ed 2, St Louis, 1997, Mosby.

Spivey WH: Intraosseous infusions, *J Pediatr* 111:639-643, 1987.

Thompson A. Pediatric emergency airway management. In Dieckmann RA, Fiser DH, Selbst SM: *Illustrated textbook of pediatric emergency and critical care procedures*, St Louis, 1997, Mosby.

Yamamoto LG: Emergency anesthesia and airway management. In Fleisher GR, Ludwig S, eds: *Textbook of pediatric emergency medicine*, ed 3, Baltimore, 1993, Williams & Wilkins, pp 65-73.

3 Mock Code Scenarios

This chapter offers 37 different life-threatening situations for resuscitation practice. The list encompasses a wide range of childhood illnesses and injuries that practitioners may be required to address at some time. Each scenario provides complete information for performing the exercise, as well as detailed progression options, expected responses, complications, and outcomes. The objectives are discussed at the end of each with additional comments on selected topics. References are provided for further study.

AIRWAY
1. Airway Obstruction—Croup
DAVID BROUSSEAU

OBJECTIVES
1. Recognize and manage upper airway obstruction.
2. Differentiate croup from other causes of upper airway obstruction.
3. Manage upper airway obstruction caused by croup.

Brief Presenting History

A 15-month-old male is carried in by his father with a chief complaint of barky cough and noisy breathing.

Initial Vital Signs

P 175, BP 95/50, RR 42.
If asked: T 37.9° C (R), estimated weight 10 kg.

Initial Physical Examination

Lying in father's arms, awake but uncomfortable appearing.
If asked:
- **Airway:** Airway patent, audible inspiratory stridor at rest.
- **Breathing:** Moderate respiratory distress with nasal congestion and flaring. Use of all accessory muscles, inspiratory stridor at rest, no rales, mild rhonchi.
- **Circulation:** Tachycardia, no murmur noted, capillary refill time 2 seconds.
- Skin: Pale, no bruises or rash.
- Mouth: Open, no drooling, mucous membranes moist, epiglottis not visualized.
- Abdomen: Soft, nontender, no masses detected.
- Neurologic: Alert, moves all extremities, very quiet.

Further History Given on Request

Three days of URI symptoms. The parents noted a barklike cough the previous evening, but the child seemed well today, eating and drinking normally. This evening respiratory distress increased. It has worsened significantly over the past hour. Low-grade temperatures only. No history of choking or foreign body ingestion.

Previous Medical History

Previously well, no medications, normal development, all immunizations received.

Expected interventions	Complications
1. Assess ABCs.	
2. Comfort the patient—allow to stay in parent's lap, minimal invasive intervention.	Vomits, requiring suctioning.
3. Humidified air or oxygen.	If agitated, develops worse stridor and cyanosis.
4. Midline head and airway positioning.	
5. Clear mouth and nose of secretions.	
6. Pulse oximeter.	Hypoxic, 90%, switch to humidified oxygen.
7. Nebulized **racemic epinephrine** 0.05 cc/kg.	
8. **Dexamethasone** 0.6 mg/kg IM.	

Progression

Initial response to racemic epinephrine nebulizer good with resolution of stridor. Soon after, however, increasing stridor, retractions, and respiratory distress develop.

Repeat Vital Signs

P 170, RR 30, pulse oximetry 88% (2 L O_2 by NC).

Expected interventions	Complications
1. Reassess ABCs.	Vomits.
2. Clear airway, suction.	Persistent respiratory distress.
3. Repeat **racemic epinephrine** nebulizer 0.05 cc/kg.	
4. Bag-valve-mask assist breaths as needed.	
5. IV access attempt.	PIV unsuccessful; consider IO.

Progression

Decreased air movement and respiratory effort noted; patient becomes somnolent.

Expected interventions	Complications
1. IO placement.	
2. Rapid sequence intubation	
No. 1.0 Miller blade.	Light does not work.
Midazolam 0.1 mg/kg IV.	
Atropine 0.02 mg/kg IV.	
Vecuronium 0.1 to 0.2 mg/kg IV.	
ETT (must have 4.0, 3.5, 3.0 ready).	Tube too large owing to swelling.
Cricoid pressure.	No cricoid pressure, vomits.
3. Place NG and end-tidal CO_2 monitor.	No NG leads to abdominal distention, vomiting, difficulty bagging.
4. CXR for ETT position.	

Repeat Vital Signs

After above resuscitation: P 150, BP 92/50, sedated with 30 bag rpm.

Additional Potential Complications

1. Progressive respiratory failure leading to hypoxia and seizure.
2. Progressive respiratory failure leading to bradycardia and cardiac arrest.
3. Right mainstem intubation or pneumothorax.

Disposition

ICU.

Discussion of Objectives

1. *Recognize and manage upper airway obstruction.*

   "A" is for airway. Initially steps must be taken to assess and manage upper airway obstruction. Assess air movement by feeling for air expelled from the mouth or nose. Listen over the airway for air movement. Watch the chest for symmetric excursion and supraclavicular muscle use.

   Inspiratory stridor is the manifestation of an extrathoracic respiratory obstruction; inspiration causes a relative negative intrathoracic pressure, which lessens the diameter of the extrathoracic airway, leading to obstruction and stridor. In croup, a viral infection, the development of airway edema exacerbates this phenomenon.

   Begin to manage an acutely obstructed airway by:

   a. Positioning the head in the midline.

   b. Using head tilt (when no trauma suspected), chin lift, and jaw thrust to prevent anatomic obstruction by structures of the hypopharynx.

   c. Suctioning the nose and mouth to clear the airway of secretions.

2. *Differentiate croup from other causes of airway obstruction.*

Other causes of upper airway obstruction include epiglottitis, foreign body aspiration, peritonsillar or retropharyngeal abscess, and bacterial tracheitis.

a. Epiglottitis—slightly older child (peak incidence 2 to 6 years) who appears "toxic." Onset is acute with high fever (usually >38.4° C), often with drooling and "sniffing position." Usually not associated with cough.

b. Foreign body aspiration—classic triad of wheezing, cough, and decreased breath sounds, no preceding URI, often a history of previous foreign body aspiration.

c. Peritonsillar or retropharyngeal abscess—asymmetry of oropharynx, often associated with toxic appearance and fever. May refuse to swallow (drooling).

d. Bacterial tracheitis—much less common, copious secretions, usually high fever (>38.4° C), frequently toxic appearing, ragged edges of the trachea seen on x-ray.

3. *Manage upper airway obstruction caused by croup.*

a. Humidified air or oxygen—mechanism not completely known (possibly moistening of secretions), but seems to work in mild cases. Avoid agitating the child because this may exacerbate stridor and respiratory distress.

b. **Dexamethasone**—no acute effects, but reduces the need for hospitalization and intubation; also decreases ICU time if necessary. PO administration appears to be as effective as IM delivery. The efficacy of inhaled, nebulized steroids is being studied.

c. **Racemic epinephrine**—nebulizer is just as effective as positive-pressure delivery; results in alpha-adrenergic vasoconstriction. No true "rebound" effect, but return of symptoms is possible after 2 to 4 hours. Dose: 0.05 cc/kg; maximum dose 0.5 cc. Some authors support discharge to home after treatment with racemic epinephrine if respiratory symptoms do not return after 3 to 4 hours of close observation. These patients should receive treatment with steroids and be able to maintain hydration.

d. Intubation—required in fewer than 1% of patients; indicated to avoid respiratory arrest. Having a smaller tube ready in case of subglottic edema is important.

REFERENCES

Bank DE, Krug SE: New approaches to upper airway disease, *Emerg Med Clin North Am* 13:473-487, 1995.

Custer JR: Croup and related disorders, *Pediatr Rev* 14:19-29, 1993.

Klassen TP et al: The efficacy of nebulized budesonide in dexamethasone-treated outpatients with croup, *Pediatrics* 97:463-466, 1996.

Ledwith C, Mauro RD: Safety and efficacy of nebulized racemic epinephrine in conjunction with oral dexamethasone and mist in the outpatient treatment of croup, *Ann Emerg Med* 25:331-337, 1995.

2. Airway Obstruction—Foreign Body Aspiration

STEPHEN J. TEACH

OBJECTIVES
1. Recognize the presentation of airway obstruction.
2. Recognize hypercarbia and hypoxia and the progression to respiratory arrest.
3. Manage acute airway obstruction and respiratory arrest.

Brief Presenting History

A 7-year-old male is brought by EMTs from Fenway Park with a chief complaint of difficulty breathing.

Initial Vital Signs

P 140, RR 40, BP 100/60.
If asked: T 37° C (R), estimated weight 25 kg.

Initial Physical Examination

General appearance: An awake, pale, diaphoretic child with severe respiratory distress.
If asked:
- **Airway:** Patent, audible inspiratory stridor.
- **Breathing:** Severe retractions and nasal flaring, breath sounds equal but diminished, no wheezing but significant stridor.
- **Circulation:** Heart tones normal, perioral cyanosis, capillary refill time 2 to 3 seconds.
- Abdomen soft and nontender with positive bowel sounds.
- No external evidence of trauma.
- Remnants of a Fenway Frank bun in mouth.

Further History Given on Request

EMTs were called to the centerfield bleachers during the fourth inning of a Red Sox–Yankees game. The child had been eating a Fenway Frank when a Red Sox player hit a screaming line drive off the wall in left. In the excitement the child choked and became abruptly short of breath. A bleacher bum attempted the Heimlich maneuver but succeeded only in getting mustard on a lady in the row in front of them.

Previous Medical History

Negative, no reactive airways disease.
No medications, NKDA.

Expected interventions	Complications
1. ABCs, look in the mouth!	
2. Attempt foreign body removal with abdominal thrusts alternating with back blows.	Unable to remove foreign body.
3. 100% O_2 by face mask.	
4. ECG monitors and oximeter.	
5. Establish IV access.	IV access unsuccessful.
6. Order portable CXR/lateral neck.	
7. Call ORL/ENT or general surgeons.	

Repeat Vital Signs

P 100, RR 20 labored, BP not obtainable, oximeter not functioning.

Progression

Becomes unresponsive, abrupt cessation of air movement, followed by respiratory arrest and increasing bradycardia.

Expected interventions	Complications
1. Attempt bag-valve-mask ventilation.	No air movement with BVM.
2. Direct laryngoscopy: Piece of a hot dog at level of vocal cords.	
3. Attempt removal with Magill forceps.	

Progression	Expected interventions
Option 1	
Foreign body (FB) removed successfully with Magill forceps, patient improves dramatically.	1. Continue O_2 and monitors.
Option 2	
Foreign body removal unsuccessful.	1. Intubation past FB required.
	2. Miller no. 2 blade, 6.0 ETT.
	3. **Atropine** 0.02 mg/kg.
	4. If needed: **Midazolam** 0.1 mg/kg IV.
	5. **Vecuronium** 0.1 to 0.2 mg/kg IV or **rocuronium** 0.6 to 1 mg/kg IV.
Vomits if no cricoid pressure applied.	6. Cricoid pressure.
	7. Place NG and end-tidal CO_2 monitor.
	8. CXR for ETT position.
Patient improves dramatically with successful intubation.	

Progression	*Expected interventions*

Option 3

FB removal unsuccessful.

1. Intubation past FB required.
2. Miller no. 2 blade, 6.0 ETT.
3. **Atropine** 0.02 mg/kg.
4. If needed: **Midazolam** 0.1 mg/kg IV.
5. **Vecuronium** 0.1 to 0.2 mg/kg IV or **rocuronium** 0.6 to 1.0 mg/kg IV.

Vomits if no cricoid pressure applied.

6. Cricoid pressure.
7. Place NG and end-tidal CO_2 monitor.
8. CXR for ETT position.

Full cardiopulmonary arrest.
   No respiratory effort.
   Asystole.

9. Intubation successful.
10. Chest compressions.
11. **Epinephrine** 1:10,000, 0.1 ml/kg IV, or **epinephrine** 1:1000, 0.1 ml/kg ETT.

Resuscitation successful.

Option 4

FB removal unsuccessful.

1. Intubation past FB required.
2. Miller 2 blade, 6.0 ETT.
3. **Atropine** 0.02 mg/kg.
4. If needed: **Midazolam** 0.1 mg/kg IV.
5. **Vecuronium** 0.1 to 0.2 mg/kg IV or **rocuronium** 0.6 to 1 mg/kg IV.

Vomits if no cricoid pressure applied.

6. Cricoid pressure.
7. *Intubation unsuccessful.*
8. Attempt BVM ventilations—minimal air movement into chest.

Full cardiopulmonary arrest.
Laryngoscopy reveals portion of hot dog now beneath the cords, foreign body occluding the trachea below the level of the true vocal cords.

9. Begin chest compressions.
10. **Epinephrine** 1:10,000, 0.1 ml/kg IV; if no response, repeat with "high-dose" **epinephrine** 1:1000, 0.1 ml/kg IV.
11. Percutaneous cricothyrotomy (see Chapter 2). 16- to 18-gauge Angiocath with connector from 3.0 ETT.
    Connect to 100% oxygen at 50 psi (15 liters per minute). Deliver intermittent bursts at a rate of approximately 20 per minute. Each burst should last about 1 second on followed by 2 seconds off.
    Use jet ventilator when available.
12. Prepare for emergency surgical creation of airway in the operating room.
13. **Normal saline** fluid bolus 20 ml/kg IV for hypotension.

Additional Potential Complications

1. Seizure secondary to hypoxia and acidosis requires **lorazepam** 0.1 mg/kg IV. Administration of lorazepam leads to respiratory depression or arrest.

Disposition

Option 1—home.
Option 2 or 3—ICU/OR for FB removal.
Option 4—OR for FB removal, possible establishment of a surgical airway.

Discussion of Objectives

1. *Recognize the presentation of airway obstruction.*
   The obvious lack of chest expansion and the audible stridor make airway obstruction likely in this patient. The differential diagnosis of stridor includes foreign body, retropharyngeal mass, epiglottitis, laryngotracheitis (croup), and extrinsic airway compression. Airway obstruction must always be considered, since it is a medical emergency of the highest priority.
2. *Recognize hypercarbia and hypoxia and the progression to respiratory arrest.*
   This patient displays evidence of decreased ventilation and oxygenation caused by poor air entry secondary to airway obstruction. Failure to gain control of the airway leads to progressive hypercarbia and hypoxia and subsequent cardiopulmonary arrest.
3. *Manage acute airway obstruction and respiratory arrest.*
   The diagnosis depends on the age of the patient, history, signs, and symptoms. Treatment of foreign body aspiration lies in attempts to move air by either removing the foreign body or providing an artificial airway around it. Initial removal attempts begin with chest thrusts (patients less than 1 year of age) or abdominal thrusts (patients greater than 1 year of age) alternating with back blows. Avoid blind finger sweeps in infants and children. If thrusts and back blows are unsuccessful, the next step is direct laryngoscopy and removal by forceps. The practitioner must be ready to circumvent the obstruction with a surgical airway (percutaneous cricothyrotomy).

Additional Comments

1. Surgical airway techniques are controversial in the pediatric population (see Chapter 2). The narrowest part of the airway in a child less than 8 years of age is the subglottic cricoid ring inferior to the cricothyroid membranes. When a foreign body is lodged at this level, cricothyrotomy may not be effective. However, cricothyrotomy should not be withheld when other methods fail to provide airway patency.

REFERENCES

Brownstein DR: Foreign bodies of the gastrointestinal tract and airway. In Barkin RM, ed: *Pediatric emergency medicine: concepts and clinical practice*, ed 2, St Louis, 1997, Mosby.

Healy GB: Management of tracheobronchial foreign bodies in children: an update, *Ann Otol Rhinol Laryngol* 99:889-891, 1990.

Mace SE: Cricothyrotomy. In Roberts JR, Hedges JR, eds: *Clinical procedures in emergency medicine*, Philadelphia, 1991, WB Saunders, pp 48-60.

3. Airway Obstruction—Anaphylaxis

ANNE M. STACK

OBJECTIVES

1. Recognize acute airway obstruction caused by anaphylaxis.
2. Appreciate the wide range of symptom severity in anaphylaxis.
3. Understand the three major mechanisms by which anaphylaxis is mediated.

Brief Presenting History

An 11-year-old female with known L-3 myelomeningocele, VP shunt, seizure disorder, and neurogenic bladder has fever, flank pain, and foul-smelling urine. She was in her usual state of health until this morning. Her mother states that this is just how she behaves when she has a urinary tract infection.

While undergoing urinary catheterization, the girl suddenly complains of tightness in the chest and a sensation that her throat is "closing in." This progresses to complaints of dizziness, and the patient becomes difficult to arouse.

Initial Vital Signs

HR 130, RR 30 with audible stridor, BP 60/25.
If asked: T 37.2° C, estimated weight 40 kg.

Initial Physical Examination

General appearance: Acute respiratory distress.
If asked: Developing widespread urticaria, swollen lips and tongue.
- **Airway:** Poor air movement, audible stridor.
- **Breathing:** Profound dyspnea, gasping for air, stridor and wheezing heard on auscultation.
- **Circulation:** Skin flushed, capillary refill time 2 to 3 seconds.
- Minimal response to painful stimulus.

Further History Given on Request

When asked, the mother states that the patient had hives before when she was in the hospital and that she had been given special urinary catheters to use at home because of "reactions" to the catheters used initially.

Expected interventions	Complications
1. Assess ABCs.	
2. Monitors (ECG/oximeter).	
3. 100% oxygen, assist with BVM.	Vomits, requires suctioning.
4. **Epinephrine** 1:1000, 0.01 ml/kg SQ; maximum dose 0.3 ml SQ.	
5. Two large-bore IVs. **Normal saline** 20 ml/kg IV.	IV access unsuccessful.
6. CVL placement.	

Repeat Vital Signs

HR 150, RR 8, BP unobtainable.

Progression	Expected interventions
Option 1 Patient becomes unresponsive. No air movement with BVM. Patient improves with intubation and epinephrine.	1. Attempt tracheal intubation with Miller no. 2 blade, 6.0 ETT. 2. **Epinephrine** 1:10,000 0.1 ml/kg IV. If no IV access, give via ETT or **epinephrine** 1:1000 0.3 ml SQ.
Option 2 Patient becomes unresponsive. No air movement with BVM. Unable to intubate because of airway edema. Patient improves with intubation and epinephrine.	1. Attempt tracheal intubation with Miller no. 2 blade, 6.0 ETT. 2. Change to 5.5 or 5.0 ETT. 3. **Epinephrine** 1:10,000 0.1 ml/kg IV. If no IV access, give **epinephrine** 1:1000 0.1 ml/kg ETT or **epinephrine** 1:1000 0.3 ml SQ. 3. **Normal saline** 20 ml/kg IV bolus. 4. Beta agonist, **albuterol** 0.5 cc. Nebulizer treatment via ETT. 5. Consider **epinephrine** 0.1 μg/kg/min continuous IV infusion.
Option 3 Patient becomes unresponsive. No air movement with BVM.	1. Attempt tracheal intubation with Miller no. 2 blade, 6.0 ETT.

Progression	Expected interventions

Option 3—cont'd

Unable to intubate because of airway edema.

2. Change to 5.5 or 5.0 ETT.
3. **Epinephrine** 1:10,000 0.1 ml/kg IV. If no IV access, give **epinephrine** 1:1000 0.1 ml/kg ETT or **epinephrine** 1:1000 0.3 ml SQ.
4. **Normal saline** 20 ml/kg IV bolus.

Still unable to intubate.

5. Perform cricothyrotomy.
6. Consider **epinephrine** 0.1 μg/kg/min continuous IV infusion.

See Cricothyrotomy in Chapter 2, p. 11.

◆

Progression

Patient improves with surgical airway.

Expected Interventions

1. **Methylprednisolone** 2 mg/kg IV.
2. **Diphenhydramine** 1 mg/kg IV.

Additional Potential Complications

1. Ventricular tachycardia or ventricular fibrillation develops, necessitating cardioversion or defibrillation.
2. Excessive delivered positive pressure leads to decreased breath sounds on the right and desaturation, i.e., tension pneumothorax.
3. A large hematoma is noted at the femoral venous CVL site, necessitating removal and replacement of the line to the opposite side.

Disposition

ICU.

Discussion of Objectives

1. *Recognize acute airway obstruction caused by anaphylaxis.*
   Anaphylactic reactions are characterized by the sudden onset of skin flushing, urticaria, and airway obstruction, leading to hypoxia and finally cardiovascular collapse.
   The rapid progression of symptoms is indicative of the severity of the reaction. Rapid institution of epinephrine may be lifesaving because it reverses laryngospasm, bronchospasm, capillary leak, vasodilation, and myocardial suppression and may inhibit further mediator release.
   Methylprednisolone and **diphenhydramine** are also used to blunt the immune-mediated and mast cell response.

2. *Appreciate the wide range of symptom severity in anaphylaxis.*

   Anaphylaxis can be initiated by any route of exposure and is most commonly caused by insect venom, drugs, and foods. In patients with myelomeningocele there is a well-described increased incidence of *latex allergy.*

   The quantity of allergen, route of exposure, and sensitivity of the patient determine the extent of the anaphylaxis event. Some patients exhibit a biphasic reaction with symptoms recurring after several hours. Patients who initially complain of airway symptoms or who demonstrate decrease in blood pressure should be admitted for observation.

3. *Understand the three major mechanisms by which anaphylaxis is mediated.*

   a. *Classic IgE-mediated:* IgE antibodies formed on initial exposure to the antigen bind to high-affinity receptors on mast cells and basophils; on reexposure the antigen induces bridging of IgE molecules leading to degranulation and release of preformed and rapidly generated histamine.

   b. Immune complexes activate the complement cascade, and *anaphylatoxins (C3a and C5a)* directly trigger release of mediators from mast cells and basophils.

   c. Certain agents may *directly stimulate release of mediators* by an unknown mechanism that does not involve IgE or complement (e.g., use of mannitol or radiocontrast media). Among the mediators responsible are histamine, prostaglandin D_2, leukotriene C4, platelet-activating factor, tryptase, and chymase.

REFERENCES

Bochner BS, Lichtenstein LM: Anaphylaxis, *N Engl J Med* 324:178-179, 1991.

Edwards KH, Johnston C: Allergic and immunologic disorders. In Barkin RM, ed: *Pediatric emergency medicine: concepts and clinical practice*, ed 2, St Louis, 1997, Mosby.

Kobrynski LJ: Latex: allergen of the '90's, *Contemp Pediatr* 13:87-95, 1996.

Kulick RM, Ruddy RM: Allergic emergencies. In Fleisher GR, Ludwig S, eds: *Textbook of pediatric emergency medicine*, ed 3, Baltimore, 1993, Williams & Wilkins, pp 858-873.

Landwehr LP, Bogniewicz M: Current perspectives on latex allergy, *J Pediatr* 128:305-312, 1996.

Sampson HA, Mendelson L, Rosen JP: Fatal and near-fatal anaphylactic reactions to food in children and adolescents, *N Engl J Med* 327:380-384, 1992.

Saryan JA, O'Loughlin JM: Anaphylaxis in children, *Pediatr Ann* 21:590-598, 1992.

4. Airway Obstruction—Tracheostomy

KATHLENE BASSETT

OBJECTIVES

1. Understand the basics of tracheostomy tubes.
2. Recognize complications associated with tracheostomy tubes.
3. Recognize alternatives to airway management with a tracheostomy tube.

Brief Presenting History

A 3-year-old tracheostomy-dependent child presents with severe respiratory distress. The tracheostomy tube appears to be in place.

Initial Vital Signs

P 180, BP 102/70, RR 68.
If asked: T 37.8, estimated weight 14 kg.

Initial Physical Examination

General appearance: The patient is agitated and cyanotic with severe retractions.
If asked: Anxious appearing.

- **Airway:** Poor air entry. Small amounts of mucus are coming from the tracheostomy tube.
- **Breathing:** Intercostal and substernal retractions, poor air movement, breath sounds significantly diminished bilaterally, occasional rhonchi, no wheezing.
- **Circulation:** Heart is tachycardic, but heart tones are difficult to hear. Capillary refill time 5 to 6 seconds.

Further History Given on Request

This child was in a motor vehicle collision several months ago, which left her neurologically devastated. She received a tracheostomy for long-term ventilation. The current tracheostomy tube has been in place for 3 months. She is ventilator dependent only at night. She became acutely short of breath tonight.

- No fever.
- Suctioning and repositioning of the cannula at home have already been attempted without improvement.
- NKDA, no medications.

Expected interventions	Complications
1. 100% oxygen to tracheostomy tube.	No improvement.
2. Suction tracheostomy tube, attempt bag ventilations.	No improvement. Difficult to bag.
3. Monitors (ECG and pulse oximeter).	
4. Attempt IV access.	IV access unsuccessful.
5. Laboratory tests: ABG.	

Progression

The child continues to have marked respiratory distress despite interventions. Suctioning the tube was unsuccessful, and bag-valve-tracheostomy breathing is difficult. Pulse oximetry is 87%.

Expected Interventions

1. Prepare to replace tracheostomy:
   Obtain a cannula of the same size or smaller, or an endotracheal tube of the same caliber.
   Place a towel under the shoulders to hyperextend the neck.
   Remove the tracheostomy tube.
   Attempt reinsertion of the cannula.
2. Notify ENT.

Progression

The stoma is very constricted, and you cannot advance the cannula. The child is extremely agitated. A small amount of bleeding has occurred at the stoma site.

Expected interventions	Complications
1. Call for assistance from ENT, surgery, or anesthesia.	
2. Place flexible oxygen tubing into the stoma, and attempt to insert the cannula over the tubing.	Unable to insert the cannula.
3. Prepare for rapid sequence intubation.	Pulse oximetry 85%.
4. BVM oral airway while covering stoma.	Patient is poorly responsive.
5. If no IV access, place IO.	
6. Rapid sequence intubation. Miller No. 2 blade, 4.5 ETT.	Unable to pass 4.5 ETT because of subglottic stenosis. Use 4.0 ETT.
Atropine 0.01 mg/kg IV/IO or **midazolam** 0.1 mg/kg IV/IO or **succinylcholine** 1 mg/kg IV/IO or **rocuronium** 0.6 to 1 mg/kg IV/IO. Cricoid pressure. Place NG tube and end-tidal CO_2 monitor. CXR to check ETT position.	Vomits if no cricoid pressure applied.
7. Laboratory tests: ABG.	

Additional Potential Complications

1. A child presents with accidental decannulation. Attempt to replace the cannula immediately.
2. Chest x-ray reveals the presence of a pneumomediastinum or pneumothorax resulting from a false tracheal passage.

Disposition

ICU.

Discussion of Objectives

1. *Understand the basics of tracheostomy tubes.*
   Tracheostomy tubes are frequently placed in patients requiring chronic mechanical ventilation. A variety of both metal and plastic tracheostomy tubes are available. Metal tracheostomy tubes consist of the tracheostomy tube and an inner cannula. Shiley and Portex plastic tubes have a single cannula and are more frequently used for long-term mechanical ventilation than metal tubes. Plastic, single-lumen tubes are preferred over metal tubes because they have a larger inner diameter and the lower surface tension of plastic keeps the tubes cleaner, resulting in less mucous plugging and obstruction. Uncuffed tracheostomy tubes are more often used in the pediatric population, although cuffed tubes are often used in older children.
2. *Recognize complications associated with tracheostomy tubes.*
   Many tracheostomy-dependent children are cared for in the home with the assistance of home health care agencies. Some of these children are ventilator dependent. The most common cause of respiratory distress associated with a tracheostomy is mechanical obstruction of the cannula, often secondary to mucous plugging. After preoxygenation, suctioning should be attempted. If the suction catheter will not pass through the tracheal cannula, it must be changed immediately. Reinsertion may cause complications, including bleeding, creation of a false tracheal passage, pneumothorax, pneumomediastinum, and rarely, perforation of the trachea. False tracheal passages occur in tissue planes outside the trachea, most commonly 7 to 10 days after tracheostomy placement. Late complications include granuloma or stricture formation at the stoma or where the tip of the tube meets the tracheal wall. An uncommon but dangerous late complication is erosion of the tracheostomy tube into the innominate artery.
   Toddlers and young children may inadvertently (or purposely!) decannulate themselves. Parents are usually able to recannulate the trachea without difficulty, but occasionally recannulation is not possible and acute respiratory distress may ensue.
3. *Recognize alternatives to airway management with a tracheostomy tube.*
   If a tracheostomy tube has become dislodged, insert a new tube of similar size or smaller or (if no other tube is available) reinsert the same tube. If no tracheostomy tube is available, use an endotracheal tube with the same diameter. The tracheal stoma may constrict and make cannula insertion difficult. A small oxygen catheter can be inserted temporarily into the stoma and used as a stylet for passage of a tracheal cannula.
   If the tracheostomy tube becomes obstructed, preoxygenate the patient with 100% oxygen and attempt to suction the tube. If you are unable to suction or the child is in significant distress, remove the tracheostomy tube. Attempt to reinsert the tracheal cannula. If insertion of a tracheal cannula is unsuccessful, attempt to insert a cannula using oxygen tubing as a stylet. If all these

measures fail, contact the surgery and anesthesia departments and prepare for oral endotracheal intubation. Bag-valve-mask the oral airway while covering the tracheal stoma in preparation for intubation. Recognize that endotracheal intubations may be difficult if the tracheostomy was placed because of anatomic airway abnormalities. Have readily available several endotracheal tubes of smaller than expected size.

REFERENCES

Arnold J: Tracheotomy. In Blumer J, ed: *A practical guide to pediatric intensive care*, ed 3, St Louis, 1990, Mosby, pp 992-993.

Ruddy RM: Procedures. In Fleisher GR, Ludwig S, eds: *Textbook of pediatric emergency medicine*, ed 3, Baltimore, 1993, Williams & Wilkins, pp 1622-1623.

Thompson AE: Pediatric airway management. In Fuhrman BP, Zimmerman JJ, eds: *Pediatric critical care*, St Louis, 1992, Mosby, pp 125-126.

Wetmore RF: Tracheotomy. In Bluestone CD, Stool SE, Kenna MA, eds: *Pediatric otolaryngology*, ed 3, Philadelphia, 1996, WB Saunders, pp 1427-1437.

BREATHING
5. Respiratory Distress—Pneumonia
KRISTINE RITTICHIER

OBJECTIVES

1. Recognize respiratory distress and impending respiratory failure.
2. Recognize the signs and symptoms of pneumonia.
3. Manage the common complications of pneumonia.
4. Recognize and treat the common causes of pneumonia.

Brief Presenting History

A 2-year-old who has had an upper respiratory infection for 1 week now presents with increased work of breathing, acute onset of fever, and increased cough.

Initial Vital Signs

P 168, BP 102/70, RR 76.
If asked: T 40.1° C (R), estimated weight 15 kg.

Initial Physical Examination

General appearance: Pale, lying in mother's arms with nasal flaring and coughing, ill appearing.
If asked:
- **Airway:** Patent.
- **Breathing:** Intercostal, subcostal, and suprasternal retractions, diminished aeration in left base, crackles and bronchial breath sounds in left middle and upper lobes.
- **Circulation:** Tachycardic without murmur, femoral pulses slightly diminished, capillary refill time 3 seconds.
- HEENT: Unremarkable except crusted nasal drainage.
- Mucous membranes dry.
- Neck: Supple without meningeal signs.
- Abdomen: Soft, nontender, no hepatosplenomegaly, bowel sounds diminished.
- Neurologic: Alert, looking around, nonfocal, anxious.

Further History Given on Request

The patient has been drinking very little and not eating. He has complained of abdominal pain and has coughed up green-yellow mucus.

Expected interventions	*Complications*
1. 100% oxygen by face mask.	No improvement with oxygen.
2. Monitors and pulse oximetry.	Pulse oximeter not reading.
3. IV access attempt.	IV access attempt unsuccessful.
4. Rapid glucose, CBC, blood culture, ABG.	
5. Call for CXR.	
6. **Acetaminophen** 15 mg/kg PR.	

Repeat Vital Signs

Pulse 178, BP 100/70, RR 63, T 39.2° C.

Laboratory Results

Rapid glucose 89, ABG: pH 7.18, P_{CO_2} 70, P_{O_2} 86 on 10 L nonrebreather mask.

Progression

The patient's respiratory rate slows to 12, pulse is 110, and he becomes unresponsive. Capillary refill time 4 to 5 seconds. Minimal breath sounds on the left.

Expected interventions	*Complications*
1. BVM-assisted breathing.	Copious secretions, vomiting.
2. IO placement.	
Normal saline 20 ml/kg.	
3. Rapid sequence intubation.	Suction not hooked to wall.
No. 1.0 Miller blade.	Laryngoscope light not working.
Atropine 0.02 mg/kg IV.	Difficulty with oxygenation secondary to right
Midazolam 0.1 mg/kg IV.	mainstem intubation or abdominal distention.
Succinylcholine 1.0 mg/kg IV.	
4.5 ETT (4.0 and 5.0 ready).	
NG tube, end-tidal CO_2 monitor.	
CXR for ETT position.	

Progression

Heart rate increases to 150 bpm, but pulse oximetry is 88%. Capillary refill time is 4 seconds. Breath sounds are minimal on the left.

Expected interventions	Complications
1. Provide positive end-expiratory pressure (PEEP).	No improvement, pulse oximeter 85%.
2. Thoracentesis, 20-gauge needle over second rib, midclavicular line.	No air from needle, small amount of fluid.
3. Chest tube placement 20 Fr over fourth rib (level of nipple) at midaxillary line.	Ineffective because of failure to hook up suction.

See Thoracentesis (p. 12) and Thoracostomy Tube (p. 13) in Chapter 2.

Progression

Large amount of yellow-green fluid expressed from chest tube. Increased breath sounds on the left. Perfusion 3 to 4 seconds.

Expected interventions	Complications
1. Repeat **normal saline** 20 ml/kg bolus IV/IO.	IO infiltrates.
2. Femoral line placement.	
3. Consider **dopamine** continuous infusion. Start at 10 µg/kg/min IV.	
4. IV **antibiotics**.	

Additional Potential Complications

1. Hypoxia caused by plug in endotracheal tube.
2. Disseminated intravascular coagulation resulting from sepsis.

Disposition

ICU.

Discussion of Objectives

1. *Recognize respiratory distress and impending respiratory failure.*
   Respiratory distress is defined as the inability to maintain gas exchange at the rate that matches the body's metabolic rate. It is evidenced as abnormal respirations, including tachypnea, bradypnea, apnea, or increased work of breathing. Use of accessory muscles, nasal flaring, grunting, cyanosis, decreased mental status, and decreased air movement on auscultation are additional signs of respiratory distress found on physical examination.
   The signs and symptoms of respiratory distress are useful for assessing the severity of illness and dictating the urgency of evaluation and therapy. The diagnosis is aided by determining oxygen saturation via pulse oximetry and arterial blood gas sample. The presence of acidosis with a P_{CO_2} greater than 50 mm Hg or a P_{O_2} less than 50 mm Hg indicates impending respiratory failure.

Oxygen therapy and cardiac monitoring should be initiated immediately for patients in respiratory distress. Intubation may be indicated for severe respiratory distress, ventilatory failure, or acidosis.

2. *Recognize the signs and symptoms of pneumonia.*

   Pneumonia is an acute infection of the lung parenychema, and classic signs include fever, cough, rales, and evidence of pulmonary consolidation on physical examination. Chest radiographic changes can lag behind the clinical presentation initially. Commonly accompanying infections include otitis media, pharyngitis, and rhinitis. Abdominal pain or ileus is often present.

3. *Manage the common complications of pneumonia.*

   Common complications of pneumonia include copious secretions, bronchospasm and wheezing, hypoxia and hypercapnia, pleural effusion, empyema, and septic shock. Support includes 100% oxygen, suctioning, nebulized beta$_2$ agonists, thoracentesis or chest tube placement, and vigorous support of perfusion with isotonic fluids and vasopressors as indicated by severity of shock.

4. *Recognize and treat the common etiologies of pneumonia.*

   In children, most lower respiratory infections (LRI), including pneumonias, are caused by viruses. The most common are respiratory syncytial virus, human parainfluenza virus, influenza virus, and adenovirus. During the child's first year of life 70% of LRI are viral in etiology, and this percentage changes to 50% at school age.

   Bacterial pneumonias usually run a more acute and virulent course. Common bacterial pathogens include *Streptococcus pneumoniae, Haemophilus influenzae,* and *Staphylococcus aureus.* Unusual organisms include *Bordetella pertussis, Chlamydia trachomatis,* and *Mycoplasma pneumoniae.* Mixed infections with both viral and bacterial pathogens have also been detected.

   Antibiotics should be initiated in patients suspected of having a bacterial illness. Even when a viral infection is suspected, antibiotics should be strongly considered until culture results are available if the patient appears "toxic" or experiences respiratory distress. The initial choice of treatment should be based on the common causes of disease for the patient's age group, the patient's allergies, and known bacterial sensitivity patterns.

REFERENCES

Henrickson K: Lower respiratory viral infections in immunocompetent children, *Adv Pediatr Infect Dis* 9:59-96, 1994.

Turner RB et al: Pneumonia in pediatric outpatients, *J Pediatr* 111:194-200, 1987.

6. Respiratory Distress—Asthma

LYDIA CIARALLO

OBJECTIVES

1. Recognize status asthmaticus and its predisposing factors.
2. Recognize impending respiratory failure.
3. Understand the general principles and inherent complications associated with intubation of an asthmatic patient.

Brief Presenting History

A 13-year-old female began wheezing 4 hours before arrival. An albuterol inhaler used at home was not helpful. Breathing is moderately labored.

Initial Vital Signs

RR 48, HR 100, BP 140/80.
If asked: T 37.4° C, estimated weight 50 kg.

Initial Physical Examination

General appearance: Patient sitting forward on bed, dyspneic, unable to complete sentences, combative when approached.
If asked:
- **Airway:** Patent.
- **Breathing:** Nasal flaring with suprasternal and intercostal retractions. Poor air movement bilaterally, barely audible tight wheezes throughout.
- **Circulation:** Tachycardic without murmur, capillary refill time 2 seconds.
- Pulse oximeter 92%.
- Peak flow 80 L/min (<50% of predicted).
- Pulsus paradoxus 15 mm Hg.

Further History Given on Request

- Chronic history of asthma, patient previously admitted to the ICU, never intubated.
- Last admission several years ago.
- Medications: Albuterol inhaler PRN only.
- NKDA, no history of anaphylaxis.
- Previously well, no antecedent URI symptoms.
- Mother believes patient may be smoking with kids at school.

Expected interventions	Complications
1. 100% oxygen by face mask.	No improvement with O_2.
2. Monitors (ECG and oximeter).	
3. IV access attempts.	
4. Nebulized **albuterol** 2.5 to 5.0 mg in 2 cc NS.	If too combative for nebulizer, give **epinephrine** 1:1000, 0.1 ml/kg SQ.
5. **Methylprednisolone** 2 mg/kg IV.	
6. ABG.	

Progression

Marked deterioration between nebulizations, decreasing respiratory effort.

Repeat Vital Signs

RR 14, HR 60, BP 100/60, pulse oximeter 88% on 6 L O_2.

Laboratory Results

ABG: pH 7.24, Pco_2 60, Po_2 80 on 6 L O_2.

Expected interventions	Complications
1. Continuous albuterol nebulization 10 to 15 mg/hr.	Vomiting, requiring suction.
2. Consider additional aggressive status asthmaticus therapies:	
Ipratropium 0.5 mg nebulizer.	
Terbutaline 4 to 10 µg/kg IV bolus over 5 to 10 minutes; 0.2 to 0.4 µg/kg/min continuous IV infusion.	
Aminophylline 6 mg/kg IV bolus; 1 mg/kg/hr continuous IV infusion.	
Magnesium 2 g slow IVP.	

Note: Acute pharmacologic management of status asthmaticus is far from standardized. Actual medications and dosages used vary among institutions and clinicians. Recognition of the need for aggressive intervention is the goal.

Progression

The patient becomes lethargic, and no air movement is audible on auscultation.

Expected interventions	Complications

1. Rapid sequence intubation.
    Preoxygenate.
    Suction.
    7.0 cuffed ETT, Mac blade no. 2 or 3.
    Atropine 0.02 mg/kg IV (before ketamine).
    Ketamine 1 to 2 mg/kg IV.
    Succinylcholine 1 to 2 mg/kg IV or
        vecuronium 0.1 to 0.2 mg/kg IV.
	Copious secretions, requires suctioning.
	
	Left mainstem intubation.

2. Auscultate for position, tape in place.	If tube is handled improperly, patient is extubated.
3. Place NG tube and end-tidal CO_2 monitor.	
4. Call for CXR to check ETT position.	

Progression

Transient improvement after intubation successfully completed, quickly followed by deteriorating condition, pulse oximeter in the low 80s, HR 50, heart tones deviated to the right, decreased breath sounds on the left.

Expected interventions	Complications
1. Recognize tension pneumothorax.	
2. Left chest thoracentesis, 18-gauge needle.	Ineffective because of improper syringe- stopcock setup.
3. Chest tube placement, 32 Fr.	Ineffective because of failure to connect chest tube to suction.

See Thoracentesis (p. 12) and Thoracostomy Tube (p. 13) in Chapter 2.

Additional Potential Complications

1. Delay in evacuation of tension pneumothorax, leading to asystole.

Disposition

ICU.

Discussion of Objectives

1. *Recognize status asthmaticus and its predisposing factors.*
   Status asthmaticus is a life-threatening form of asthma that accounts for most deaths resulting from this disease. It is defined as a progressively severe asthma attack that is unresponsive to the usual appropriate therapy with adrenergic drugs and that leads to disabling acute pulmonary insufficiency.

Cough, dyspnea, and wheezing are the major clinical features of status asthmaticus. The degree of wheezing does not correlate well with the severity of the attacks, but the relative absence of wheezing in the presence of respiratory distress and poor air entry on auscultation of the lungs are indicative of severe obstruction. The use of accessory muscles of respiration and the presence of pulsus paradoxus (>18 mm Hg in adolescents, >10 mm Hg in children) usually signify severe compromise of respiratory function.

2. *Recognize impending respiratory failure.*

A clinical scoring system exists to detect an impending or existing respiratory failure in patients with status asthmaticus based on the signs and symptoms of airway obstruction, use of accessory respiratory muscles, oxygenation, and cerebral function (Table 3-1).

Table 3-1   *Clinical Scoring System for Respiratory Failure in Status Asthmaticus*

	Score		
Variable	**0**	**1**	**2**
Pao_2	70-100 in air	≤70 in air	≤70 in 40% O_2
Cyanosis	None	In air	In 40% O_2
Inspiratory breath sounds	Normal	Unequal	Decreased to absent
Accessory muscles used	None	Moderate	Maximal
Expiratory wheezing	None	Moderate	Marked
Cerebral function	Normal	Depressed or agitated	Coma

From Wood DW, Downes JJ, Leeks HI: *Am J Dis Child* 123:227, 1972.

Additional features of impending respiratory failure include hypercapnia with a Pco_2 greater than 40 mm Hg in the presence of dyspnea and wheezing, metabolic acidosis, and ECG abnormalities.

Patients who have the following clinical signs and therapeutic requirements that suggest respiratory failure may require admission to the ICU:

a. Impending or existing respiratory failure as assessed by an asthma score greater than 5.
b. Terbutaline infusion.
c. Respiratory or cardiac arrest.
d. Mechanical ventilation.

3. *Understand the general principles and inherent complications associated with intubation of an asthmatic patient.*

A small number of children, despite recent advances in the pharmacologic management of status asthmaticus, develop rapidly progressive respiratory failure, resulting in coma and death. The most effective treatment of respiratory failure in these children is ventilatory support through mechanical ventilation to reduce the work of breathing and allow the bronchodilating drugs to act. No absolute guidelines have been laid down for initiating mechanical ventilation in status asthmaticus, except cardiopulmonary arrest and coma. However, the criteria that should be considered, assuming the patient has received maximal therapy including a terbutaline infusion, include:

a. A decrease in effective respiratory effort because of progressive exhaustion.

b. Significant deterioration in mental status.

c. Cyanosis on 40% oxygen.

d. Hypoxemia with a Po_2 less than 60 mm Hg on 100% O_2.

e. Hypercapnia with a Pco_2 greater than 60 mm Hg.

Once the patient with asthma is intubated, the course may be further complicated by pneumothoraces or pulmonary edema. Very high airway resistance exists because of severe bronchoconstriction and mucosal edema. To minimize the occurrence of pneumothorax, peak inspiratory pressure (PIP) must be given judiciously during bag ventilation, with an inspiratory/expiratory ratio of 1:2 or greater. A chest tube tray should be kept at the bedside of an intubated asthmatic patient.

The more negative intrapleural pressure during severe asthma attacks favors fluid accumulation in the interstitial spaces and around bronchioles. Providing positive end-expiratory pressure (PEEP) with ventilation may minimize this complication.

Additional Comments

1. Ketamine is considered the induction agent of choice in asthma because of its bronchodilating effects. It must be given with atropine or glycopyrrolate, since it increases secretions. Ketamine has been associated with emergence reactions, although less frequently in the pediatric population.

2. Pulsus paradoxus may be difficult to recognize in an acutely ill asthmatic patient, but a decrease greater than 20 mm Hg between normal expiration systolic blood pressure and a second blood pressure measured at the point where the Korotkoff sounds cease to disappear with inspiration indicates moderate to severe airway obstruction.

REFERENCES

Guidelines for the diagnosis and management of asthma, Expert Panel Report of the National Asthma Education Program and the National Heart, Lung, and Blood Institutes, August 1991.

Kulick RM, Ruddy RM: Allergic emergencies. In Fleisher GR, Ludwig S, eds: *Textbook of pediatric emergency medicine,* Baltimore, 1993, Williams & Wilkins, pp 858-867.

Letourneau MA, Schuh S, Gausche M: Respiratory disorders. In Barkin RM, ed: *Pediatric emergency medicine: concepts and clinical practice,* ed 2, St Louis, 1997, Mosby.

Nichols DG: Emergency management of status asthmaticus in children, *Pediatr Ann* 25:394-400, 1996.

Wood DW, Downes JJ, Leeks HI: A clinical scoring system for the diagnosis of respiratory failure, *Am J Dis Child* 123:227, 1972.

7. Respiratory Distress—Coarctation of the Aorta
LEWIS R. FIRST AND MARK G. ROBACK

OBJECTIVES
1. Recognize acute respiratory distress and altered mental status in an infant.
2. Manage acute respiratory distress and altered mental status in an infant.
3. Acutely manage a ductal-dependent cardiac lesion.

Brief Presenting History

A 2-week-old infant was brought in by parents who found him in his crib having difficulty breathing.

Initial Vital Signs

HR 180, BP 50/P right arm, RR 80.
If asked: T 38.0° C (R), estimated weight 4 kg.

Initial Physical Examination

General appearance: Lethargic, pale, mottled infant with blue lips.
If asked: Minimally responsive to painful stimulus.
- **Airway:** Patent, infant cries intermittently.
- **Breathing:** Lung fields with bilateral crackles.
- **Circulation:** Muffled heart tones, weak radial pulses, no femoral pulses, capillary refill time 3 to 4 seconds. Mottling, worse below the waist.
- Sunken fontanel.
- Pupils dilated, sluggishly responsive.
- Abdomen soft, liver palpated 3 cm below the right costal margin.

Further History Given on Request

Full-term product of an uncomplicated pregnancy, NSVD. Went home with Mom. Doing well until 5 days ago when poor feeding began. Vomiting over last several days. Decreased number of wet diapers.

Expected interventions	Complications
1. 100% O_2.	Vomits, requiring suction.
2. Monitors (ECG, oximeter).	
3. IV access attempts.	IV attempt unsuccessful, necessitating IO placement.
4. IV/IO access. **Normal saline** 20 ml/kg IV/IO.	
5. Laboratory tests: Rapid glucose, ABG, CBC, electrolytes, blood culture.	
6. Place Foley catheter, send UA/UC.	

Initial Laboratory Results

Rapid glucose 20, ABG: pH 7.03, P_{CO_2} 30, P_{O_2} 45, HCO_3 4.

Repeat Vital Signs

HR 60, BP not obtainable, RR 12.

Progression

Patient's condition progresses rapidly to asystole and total cardiopulmonary collapse.

Expected interventions	*Complications*
1. Bag-valve-mask ventilation with 100% O_2, cricoid pressure.	Vomits if no cricoid pressure.
2. Initiation of cardiac compressions.	Chest compressions ineffective if patient not on a hard board.
3. Prepare for rapid sequence intubation.	
4. **Epinephrine** 1:10,000, 0.1 ml/kg IV/IO.	
5. $D_{10}W$ 5 to 10 ml/kg or $D_{25}W$ 2 to 4 ml/kg IV/IO.	Seizure if no glucose given.
6. Rapid sequence intubation with 3.5 ETT, Miller no. 1 blade.	Ventricular fibrillation develops.
7. **Defibrillate** at 2 joules/kg. **Epinephrine** 1:1000, 0.1 ml/kg IV/IO. Repeat **defibrillation** at 4 joules/kg.	Persistent ventricular fibrillation.
8. Place NG tube, end-tidal CO_2 monitor.	If no NG is placed, vomiting and abdominal distention develop.
9. CXR to check ETT position. (See Appendix E, p. 218.)	

Radiographs

Large heart, lung fields with diffuse reticular pattern, ETT at the carina.

Expected Interventions

1. Start **prostaglandin E** 0.05 to 0.1 μg/kg/min IV/IO.
2. Recheck rapid serum glucose.
3. Pull ETT back 1 cm.
4. Consult the cardiology department.

Additional Potential Complications

1. Unexplained desaturation—development of pulmonary edema leading to increasing difficulty bagging after intubation. Initially the team is required to check mechanical sources, ETT placement, and oxygen tubing connections. Add PEEP, and consider reintubation.
2. Persistent hypotension—consider the addition of continuous inotrope infusion.
   Dobutamine 10 to 20 μg/kg/min or

Epinephrine 0.1 to 1 µg/kg/min or
Dopamine 3 to 10 µg/kg/min.

Disposition

ICU; if the patient's condition is stable, consider the cardiac catheterization laboratory.

Discussion of Objectives

1. *Recognize acute respiratory distress and altered mental status in an infant.*
   Presentation of tachypnea, cyanosis, and altered mental status must be regarded as an emergency situation needing aggressive evaluation and treatment. Causes to be considered in the neonatal period include a primarily pulmonary disease (i.e., pneumonia, bronchiolitis), septic or cardiogenic shock, severe dehydration, or a metabolic derangement such as hypoglycemia. Nonaccidental trauma is always part of the differential diagnosis of an infant in shock with altered mental status.

2. *Manage acute respiratory distress and altered mental status in an infant.*
   ABCs—attention must initially be given to the airway to assess patency and air entry. The patient is given 100% oxygen, and monitors, including a pulse oximeter, are placed. Assist breathing with bag-valve-mask ventilation as required. Heart rate less than 100 beats/min with hypotension in the newborn period is responded to by initiation of cardiac compressions.
   As the patient's condition deteriorates, the transition to advanced life support techniques with endotracheal intubation, resuscitation medications, and defibrillation is provided as indicated. Hypoglycemia is treated with 10% or 25% **dextrose** to deliver 0.5 to 1 g/kg.

3. *Acutely manage a ductal-dependent cardiac lesion.*
   Development of cardiac failure in this case is related to aortic stricture with or without hypoplasia located proximal to the patent ductus arteriosus (PDA). The preductal coarctation of the aorta leads to a right-to-left shunt through the PDA. As the ductus closes early in infancy, the amount of blood delivered to the pulmonary vascular bed is increased, leading to right-sided congestive heart failure. This patient displayed classic findings of coarctation of the aorta with loss of femoral pulses and diminished lower extremity perfusion. Right-sided heart failure is illustrated by crackles on lung examination and hepatomegaly.
   Treatment requires "reopening" the PDA by using **prostaglandin E**. The major side effect of prostaglandin E is apnea. If the patient does not require intubation for resuscitation initially, addition of prostaglandin E may lead to apnea, necessitating intubation. Patients to be transferred to another facility typically require prophylactic intubation.

Additional Comments

1. Recognition of hypoglycemia in an infant with poor feeding and vomiting treated with **glucose** 0.5 to 1 g/kg IV, typically as $D_{10}W$ 5 to 10 ml/kg or $D_{25}W$ 2 to 4 ml/kg IV/IO.
2. Blood pressure difference between upper and lower extremities is the major diagnostic feature of coarctation of the aorta. Blood pressure higher in the arms than in the legs by 20 mm Hg or more is considered significant. When the patient is in cardiac failure, blood pressure differences between the arms and legs may be minimal because of reduced cardiac output.

3. The typical auscultatory findings, aortic thrill at the suprasternal notch and II-III/VI ejection murmur along the sternal border, at the apex, and between the scapulae, may be absent or muffled because of cardiac failure.

4. Typically, congestive heart failure develops during infancy in 10% of patients with coarctation of the aorta.

5. For infants presenting with cyanosis and in a more stable condition, an ABG should be performed with and without 100% oxygen to aid in the diagnosis of cardiac lesions that allow mixture of blood from the pulmonary and cardiac circulations. (Admixture lesions will not raise PO_2 with the addition of 100% O_2.)

REFERENCES

Moller JH: Coarctation of the aorta. In *Essentials of pediatric cardiology*, ed 2, Philadelphia, 1978, FA Davis, pp 88-94.

Morriss MJH, McNamara DG: Coarctation of the aorta. In Garson AJ, Bricker JT, McNamara DG, eds: *The science and practice of pediatric cardiology*, Philadelphia, 1990, Lea & Febiger, pp 614-618.

Schamberger MS: Cardiac emergencies in children, *Pediatr Ann* 25:339-344, 1996.

8. Respiratory Distress—Diabetic Ketoacidosis

MARK G. ROBACK AND STEPHEN J. TEACH

> *OBJECTIVES*
> 1. Recognize respiratory distress as a presenting sign of diabetic ketoacidosis (DKA).
> 2. Carry out initial management of DKA.
> 3. Manage increased intracranial pressure in DKA.

Brief Presenting History

A 4-year-old male brought in by his mother has had increased work of breathing in the last 2 days but is much worse today. He has a history of reactive airways disease (RAD) but has had no response to his albuterol inhaler today.

Initial Vital Signs

P160, RR 54, BP 70/50.
If asked: T 37.6° C (ax), estimated weight 16 kg.

Initial Physical Examination

General appearance: Respiratory distress.
If asked: No evidence of head trauma.
- **Airway:** Patent.
- **Breathing:** Deep, labored respirations, using all accessory muscles. Expiratory phase not prolonged, lungs clear bilaterally without wheeze.
- **Circulation:** Heart tones normal but tachycardic, capillary refill time 3 to 4 seconds.
- Pupils 4 mm, sluggishly reactive.
- Fruity odor to breath.
- Abdomen nondistended and soft.

Further History Given on Request

A 4-pound weight loss over the last 2 weeks, drinking and urinating more than usual, no fever, URI symptoms, or complaints of pain.
- Past medical history: RAD otherwise negative.
- Medications: Albuterol inhaler only.
- NKDA.

Expected interventions	Complications
1. 100% O_2 by face mask.	
2. Monitors (ECG/oximeter).	
3. Attempt IV access.	IV access unsuccessful.
4. Rapid glucose, ABG, electrolytes.	

Repeat Vital Signs

P 152, RR 16, BP 80/60, pulse oximeter 90%.

Progression

Increasingly less responsive, respirations become agonal.

Laboratory Results

Rapid glucose >500, ABG: pH 7.0, Pco_2 16, Po_2 80, HCO_3 8.

Expected interventions	Complications
1. IO placement. **Normal saline** 20 ml/kg IV bolus.	Vomiting, requires suction.
2. Rapid sequence intubation. Miller no. 2 blade, 5.0 ETT. **Atropine** 0.02 mg/kg IV. **Midazolam** 0.1 mg/kg IV. **Succinylcholine** 1 to 2 mg/kg IV or **vecuronium** 0.1 to 0.2 mg/kg IV.	Unable to visualize cords if not properly suctioned.
Cricoid pressure. Place NG and end-tidal CO_2 monitor.	Emesis if no cricoid pressure.
Call for CXR for ETT position.	No NG results in abdominal distention and impaired ventilation.
3. Repeat ABG. 4. **Regular insulin** 0.1 unit/kg/hr continuous IV infusion. 5. Additional laboratory results: calcium, phosphorus, magnesium.	

Additional Potential Complications

1. Unequal dilated pupils or other evidence of increased intracranial pressure develops, necessitating hyperventilation and reassessment of fluid management.

Disposition

ICU for continued management of dehydration, ketoacidosis, possible increased intracranial pressure, and hypovolemia.

Discussion of Objectives

1. *Recognize respiratory distress as a presenting sign of diabetic ketoacidosis.*
   The patient in this scenario presents with signs and symptoms of ketoacidosis, including Kussmaul breathing, ketotic breath, and altered mental status. Manage respiratory distress initially with assessment of a patent airway and effective ventilation. The patient is given 100% oxygen. This patient has a history of RAD, but despite being in respiratory distress, does not

have impaired air entry, a prolonged expiratory phase, or expiratory wheezes that would be expected with a RAD exacerbation.

Further history of polyuria, polydipsia, and weight loss despite hyperphagia evident over a period of days to weeks, as well as a rapid glucose determination, confirms the diagnosis of DKA. Symptoms frequently are precipitated by an intercurrent illness, typically a mild infection, which may confuse the picture. Abdominal pain with distention and guarding, hyperpnea, and enuresis may be confused with an acute abdomen, pneumonia, or a behavioral disorder.

2. *Initial management of diabetic ketoacidosis.*

   The goals of therapy in DKA include:

   a. Correct dehydration.

   b. Reverse acidosis and ketosis.

   c. Restore normoglycemia and correction of electrolyte abnormalities.

   d. Avoid complications of therapy.

   Patients presenting in DKA typically are very dehydrated (5% to 15%). Isotonic fluids are indicated in all cases, and more aggressive fluid resuscitation may be necessary to reverse hypotension. An initial 20 ml/kg **normal saline** bolus over the first hour is typically recommended, with slow replacement of the remaining fluid deficit over the next 24 to 48 hours. Overzealous replacement of fluid deficit should be avoided, since this may precipitate cerebral edema. Patients must be closely monitored for headache, change in level of consciousness, vomiting, bradycardia, and hypertension.

   Replacing vascular volume is essential to improving tissue perfusion and acidosis.

   A continuous infusion of **regular insulin** 0.08 to 0.1 unit/kg/hr is usually required along with frequent (typically every hour) monitoring of glucose and electrolyte levels.

   Patients with DKA usually have depletion of total body potassium, and therefore potassium should be added to IV fluids after the initial normal saline bolus.

   The use of **sodium bicarbonate** to treat acidosis in DKA remains controversial and is usually reserved for patients with an initial arterial pH of less than 7.20.

3. *Management of increased intracranial pressure in DKA.*

   Increased intracranial pressure (ICP) and DKA—the etiology of this devastating complication of DKA is poorly understood. It is most likely a result of both the underlying pathophysiology of DKA and management by IV fluid resuscitation.

   The incidence of increased ICP in DKA is less than 1%. It is more common in younger diabetics and in the case of the initial presentation of new diabetics.

   The best treatment for increased ICP in DKA is prevention. The emergency department physician must watch patients with DKA closely for changes in consciousness or responsiveness that may signal the onset of increased ICP. The fluid management of these patients must be meticulously monitored. See section on increased intracranial pressure in Chapter 4 (p. 196).

REFERENCES

Hale DE: Endocrine emergencies. In Fleisher GR, Ludwig S, eds: *Textbook of pediatric emergency medicine*, ed 3, Baltimore, 1993, Williams & Wilkins, pp 940-944.

Harris GD et al: Minimizing the risk of brain herniation during treatment of diabetic ketoacidemia: a retrospective study, *J Pediatr* 117:22-31, 1990.

Klekamp J, Churchwell KB: Diabetic ketoacidosis in children: initial clinical assessment and treatment, *Pediatr Ann* 26:387-393, 1996.

Rosenbloom A: Intracerebral crises during treatment of diabetic ketoacidosis, *Diabetes Care* 13:22-33, 1990.

Saladino RA: Endocrine and metabolic disorders. In Barkin RM, ed: *Pediatric emergency medicine: concepts and clinical practice*, ed 2, St Louis, 1997, Mosby.

Sperling MA: Diabetic ketoacidosis in children. In Lebovitz HE, ed: *Therapy for diabetes mellitus and related disorders*, Falls Church, Va, 1991, American Diabetes Association, pp 36-43.

9. Apnea—Bronchiolitis

CHARLES MACIAS

OBJECTIVES

1. Recognize respiratory distress and impending respiratory failure.
2. Acutely manage apnea and respiratory failure.
3. Recognize the association of apnea with bronchiolitis.

Brief Presenting History

A 3-month-old female, born at 30 weeks' gestational age, presents with a 2-day history of cough, nasal congestion, and "funny" breathing.

Initial Vital Signs

HR 198, RR 80, BP 90/54, T 38° C (R).
If asked: Estimated weight 3 kg.

Initial Physical Examination

General appearance: Pale, thin, ill-appearing infant.
If asked: Sunken eyes, tacky mucous membranes.
- **Airway:** Patent, thick rhinorrhea, and nasal congestion.
- **Breathing:** Marked intercostal retractions, nasal flaring, and abdominal excursions. Lungs have good air movement but coarse rhonchi and scattered expiratory wheezes throughout the lung fields.
- **Circulation:** Heart has a regular but fast rate without murmurs or gallops. Capillary refill time is 3 seconds.
- Abdomen is soft and nontender.

Further History Given on Request

The mother states that within the last 6 hours the child has had two episodes in which she stopped crying, her face turned blue, and her chest stopped moving. The episodes lasted 30 seconds and resolved when the mother picked up the child.

Expected interventions	Complications
1. Assess ABCs.	Vomits formula.
2. Oxygen, suction.	
3. Monitors (ECG, pulse oximeter).	
4. Obtain IV access.	IV access unsuccessful; consider IO placement.
Normal saline 20 ml/kg IV.	
Measure rapid serum glucose.	
5. Suction nose.	

Progression

Patient becomes apneic.

Repeat Vital Signs

HR 90, RR 0, pulse oximeter 70%.

Progression	Expected interventions	Complications
Option 1		
Patient becomes responsive with stimulation. Patient continues to breathe spontaneously but with retractions and wheezes.	1. Assist breathing with BVM and 100% O_2. 2. Prepare for rapid sequence intubation. 3. Continue O_2. 4. **Albuterol** 0.25 cc by nebulizer.	Intermittent periods of apnea.
Option 2		
Patient becomes responsive with stimulation but has tachypnea and retractions. Pulse oximetry 86% during O_2.	1. Assist breathing with BVM and 100% O_2. 2. IV or place IO. 3. Rapid sequence intubation. Miller no. 0 blade, 3.5 ETT. **Atropine** 0.02 mg/kg (min 0.1 mg) IV. **Midazolam** 0.1 mg/kg IV. $+/-$ **Vecuronium** 0.1 to 0.2 mg/kg IV. Cricoid pressure.	Persistent apneic episodes. Unable to see cords because of secretions, suction. HR 40 if **atropine** not used. Vomits if no cricoid pressure.
HR 145, pulse oximetry 97% with intubation.	End-tidal CO_2 monitor, call for CXR. 4. **Albuterol** 0.25 cc nebulizer.	
Option 3		
Patient does not respond to stimulation, becomes asystolic.	1. BVM with 100% O_2. 2. Chest compressions. 3. Rapid sequence intubation with Miller no. 0 blade, 3.5 ETT. **Epinephrine** 0.1 ml/kg, 1:10,000 IV. Cricoid pressure. End-tidal CO_2 monitor, call for CXR.	No pulses with compressions if patient not on a hard surface. Unable to see cords due to secretions, suction. Vomits if no cricoid pressure.

Progression	Expected interventions	Complications
Option 3—cont'd		
Intubation successful, HR 0.	4. Continue chest compressions.	
	5. **Epinephrine** 0.1 ml/kg, 1:1000 IV.	No breath sounds on the right.
	6. Right needle thoracentesis.	
Rush of air produced.		
HR 146, pulse oximetry 90%, wheezing present.	7. Place right-sided chest tube.	Reaccumulation of pneumo-thorax if chest tube
	8. **Albuterol** 0.25 cc by nebulizer.	handled improperly or not placed.

◆

Additional Potential Complications

1. The patient may continue to manifest evidence of mild to profound dehydration because of her increased work of breathing, increased metabolic rate, and decreased ability to maintain adequate fluid intake from a markedly elevated respiratory rate. This may be manifested as hypovolemic shock. Fluid resuscitation is required.

Disposition

ICU.

Discussion of Objectives

1. *Recognize respiratory distress and impending respiratory failure.*
   Signs and symptoms of respiratory distress are varied, depending primarily on the patient's age and stage in the evolution of respiratory failure. Older children may complain of shortness of breath, chest pain, or air hunger that a preverbal child would be unable to communicate and might manifest only as "fussiness."
   The infant younger than 4 months of age is an obligate nose breather. Upper respiratory infections may therefore cause significant compromise. Attention should be given to the degree of tachypnea (the initial mechanism for preserving minute ventilation), adequacy of tidal volume (by observing chest rise or abdominal excursion), and presence of bilateral breath sounds (assessing symmetry and air movement), nasal flaring, retractions (subcostal, intercostal, supraclavicular), accessory use of neck muscles, head bobbing, and changes in inspiratory/expiratory ratio.
   Progression from respiratory distress to respiratory failure may be evident because of clinical findings of decreased or absent breath sounds, severe retractions, use of accessory muscles, cyanosis (excluding patients with cyanotic congenital heart disease), poor muscle tone, grunting, weak cough or gag, and eventual depression of mental status and response to pain.
   Physiologic findings consistent with respiratory failure include Pao_2 less than 60 mm Hg in 60% oxygen (excluding patients with cyanotic heart disease), $Paco_2$ greater than 60 mm Hg and rising, vital capacity less than 15 ml/kg, and maximum inspiratory force (pressure) greater than

-20 cm H_2O. The diagnosis of respiratory failure is based primarily on clinical parameters, and radiographs or laboratory studies should not delay a decision to secure an airway or assist ventilations. See Respiratory Distress in Chapter 4 (p. 190).

2. *Acutely manage apnea and respiratory failure.*

Management goals for the treatment of respiratory failure and apnea are the same: restoration of adequate oxygenation and ventilation. Maximizing the airway's potential to allow air flow to the lungs (i.e., by basic airway positioning maneuvers) is important. Oxygen should be delivered in the highest possible concentration to maximize tissue oxygenation, and humidification added as soon as practical. Noninvasive pulse oximetry should be monitored continuously, as should end-tidal CO_2, if available. Arterial blood gas measurement may serve as a more accurate analysis of ventilation and oxygenation.

The apneic child is only minutes from profound hypoxemia, cardiovascular collapse, and irreparable damage to the central nervous system. Any child with a definite history of apnea must be managed with caution and in a hospital setting that has sufficient resources and staff to provide respiratory resuscitation. Although stimulation may produce temporary resolution of apnea, more aggressive management is usually necessary; assisted ventilation must be provided if spontaneous ventilation is inadequate (bag-valve-mask or endotracheal tube intubation). Once endotracheal intubation has occurred, chest wall rise, symmetry of breath sounds, condensation in the endotracheal tube, absence of gastric breath sounds (in the older child), and chest radiograph must be assessed to ensure proper tube placement. See Airway (p. 9) in Chapter 2.

3. *Recognize the association of apnea with bronchiolitis.*

Although a precise definition for bronchiolitis has not been universally accepted, it may be thought of as a wheezing-associated illness in early life preceded by signs and symptoms of an upper respiratory infection. In the Northern Hemisphere it is a seasonal disease that has peak activity during the winter months and usually lasts into the spring. Serious cases occur most commonly in infants younger than 1 year, especially in the 1- to 3-month age group. Although any number of viruses (parainfluenza, influenza type A, adenovirus, rhinovirus) may cause bronchiolitis, its pathology and epidemiology are closely affiliated with those of respiratory syncytial virus (RSV), the most common cause of bronchiolitis.

Apnea is the most frequent complication of RSV infection in young infants, occurring in about 20% of hospitalized babies. Those at highest risk for apnea are extremely young, premature infants, especially those less than 44 weeks post conception.

The prognosis is good, since apnea is usually of short duration and does not tend to recur with subsequent respiratory infections. Apnea typically appears only in the initial phase of illness. Severe complications can, however, occur in children of any age with underlying cardiac or pulmonary disease or in those who are immunocompromised.

As with any infant in respiratory distress, hydration status should be evaluated and appropriate fluid therapy delivered.

Additional Comments

The use of beta$_2$ agonists such as nebulized **albuterol** may provide some aid in treating the hyperreactive airways that may accompany bronchiolitis. Although subjects in several double-blind placebo-controlled trials have shown a clinical response to nebulized albuterol, the response is not universal. Since the potential for clinically significant improvement exists, any child with bronchiolitis that causes distress should receive a trial of beta agonist therapy and subsequent therapy guided by his or her response to that trial. Nebulized anticholinergic agents do not appear to be useful in patients with bronchiolitis, while the use of nebulized **epinephrine** remains controversial.

REFERENCES

Baren JM, Seidel JS: Emergency management of respiratory distress and failure. In Barkin RM, ed: *Pediatric emergency medicine: concepts and clinical practice*, St Louis, 1997, Mosby, pp 95-103.

Hall CB: Respiratory syncytial virus: what we know now, *Cont Pediatr* 1993, pp 92-110.

Thompson AE: Respiratory distress. In Fleisher GR, Ludwig S, eds: *Textbook of pediatric emergency medicine*, ed 3, Baltimore, 1993, Williams & Wilkins, pp 450-455.

Welliver JR, Welliver RC: Bronchiolitis, *Pediatr Rev* 14:134-139, 1993.

10. Apnea—Oversedation

KAREN GRUSKIN

OBJECTIVES

1. Recognize apnea as a presentation of drug overdose.
2. Recognize and manage respiratory insufficiency and failure.
3. Manage overdoses of narcotics and benzodiazepines with specific antidotes.

Brief Presenting History

A somnolent 6-year-old is in an examining room after casting of a broken arm. The pulse oximeter alarm is beeping, and the pulse oximeter is reading 85%.

Initial Vital Signs

P 80, BP 60/30, RR 10.
If asked: T 37.5° C (R), estimated weight 20 kg.

Initial Physical Examination

General appearance: Pale, limp with perioral cyanosis.
If asked: Pinpoint pupils, unresponsive.
- **Airway:** Patent.
- **Breathing:** Shallow respirations, breath sounds clear.
- **Circulation:** Heart tones normal, capillary refill time 3 to 4 seconds.
- Abdomen soft and nontender.
- Right arm in long arm cast.
- Left arm with an IV that has blood backed up in it.

Further History Given on Request

The patient injured his arm by falling on an outstretched hand at the playground. The fall was witnessed. No head trauma, no LOC, no other injuries.
- The patient received IV sedation (**morphine** and **midazolam**) for the procedure.
- Ate dinner 1 hour ago.
- No significant past medical history.
- No routine medications, no known drug allergies.

Expected interventions	Complications
1. 100% oxygen.	O_2 tubing improperly connected. Patient remains cyanotic.
2. Monitors (ECG, oximeter).	
3. **Naloxone** 0.1 mg/kg IV/IM.	IV not functioning.
4. Attempt IV access.	
5. **Flumazenil** 0.2 mg IV/IM.	Unable to start peripheral IV.

Repeat Vital Signs

P 80, BP 50/P, RR 8. ECG monitor: bradycardia, sinus rhythm. Pulse oximeter not picking up.

Expected interventions	Complications
1. BVM ventilation with 100% O_2. 2. Suction.	Vomiting.

Progression

No response to needle sticks; shallow respirations no longer apparent.

Expected interventions	Complications
1. Continue BVM with 100% O_2. 2. Repeat **naloxone** 2 mg IV/IM and **flumazenil** 0.3 mg IM/IV.	Emesis caused by bag/mask if no cricoid pressure used. No response to medications.

Progression

Patient either responds to BVM and naloxone/flumazenil *or* remains unresponsive and becomes apneic.

Expected interventions	Complications

1. Rapid sequence intubation.
   100% oxygen.
   Atropine 0.02 mg/kg IV.
   Miller no. 2 blade.
   5.5 ETT.
   Cricoid pressure.
   Place NG and end-tidal CO_2 monitor.
   Call for CXR to check ETT position.
2. **Naloxone** 2 mg IM/IV, repeating dose every 2 to 3 minutes.
   Flumazenil 0.2 mg IM/IV, repeating dose at 1-minute intervals to maximum of 1 mg.
3. IV access if not obtained previously.
4. Volume resuscitation.
   Normal saline 20 ml/kg IV.
5. Consider **naloxone** and/or **flumazenil** continuous IV infusion.
	Unable to visualize cords because of emesis or secretions.
	
	Nonfunctioning light bulb on blade.
	
	Vomits if no cricoid pressure or if NG not placed.
	Right mainstem intubation.

Repeat Vital Signs

After above resuscitation: P 100, BP 80/50, RR 10 to 14.

Additional Potential Complications

1. Aspiration of abdominal contents, resulting in difficulty in oxygenation and ventilation.
2. If airway not properly secured, progressive respiratory failure followed by cardiac arrest caused by hypoxia or acidosis or both.
3. Seizure resulting from hypoxia or primary drug toxicity.

Disposition

ICU for ongoing management of narcotic or benzodiazepine overdose and respiratory insufficiency.

Discussion of Objectives

1. *Recognize apnea as a presentation of drug overdose.*

   The triad of coma, pinpoint pupils, and depressed respirations in a patient receiving intravenous narcotics for an orthopedic procedure should be considered narcotic overdose until proven otherwise. Administration of a benzodiazepine alone may further heighten the respiratory suppressive effects of a narcotic.

2. *Recognize and manage respiratory insufficiency and failure.*

   The initial depressed respiratory drive should be managed with 100% oxygen and ventilation assisted by bag-valve-mask as needed. Intubation may be necessary in a drug overdose in which the respiratory drive and airway protective reflexes are depressed. However, BVM assistance for several minutes until the effects of **naloxone** and **flumazenil** are apparent is often sufficient. Patients with an initial good response to the above drugs may require additional doses to prevent relapse into somnolence and respiratory depression.

3. *Manage overdoses of narcotics and benzodiazepines with specific antidotes.*

   Narcotic overdoses can be treated with **naloxone** 0.1 mg/kg IV/IM/ETT (approximately 1 mg for a young child, 2 mg for school-age children and older). Repeat every 2 to 5 minutes as needed up to a total dose of 10 to 20 mg. Be aware that naloxone can precipitate an abstinence syndrome in patients with chronic narcotic use.

   Benzodiazepine overdoses can be treated with **flumazenil** as follows: Infant (<6 months old): 0.02 mg/kg (up to 0.2 mg) IV over 15 seconds; may be repeated every 45 seconds up to a maximum dose of 1 mg in the first hour. Pediatric/adult (>6 months old): 0.2 mg IV over 15 seconds, followed 45 seconds later by 0.3 mg, followed 45 seconds later by 0.5 mg up to a maximum dose of 3 mg. Flumazenil is contraindicated for patients receiving benzodiazepine for status epilepticus or chronic benzodiazepine therapy for a seizure disorder, as well as after acute tricyclic antidepressant ingestions.

   If frequent repeated doses are necessary, both drugs can be administered as continuous infusions.

REFERENCES

Committee on Drugs: Guidelines for monitoring and management of pediatric patients during and after sedation for diagnostic and therapeutic procedures, *Pediatrics* 89:1110-1114, 1992.

Cote CJ: Sedation for the pediatric patient, *Pediatr Clin North Am* 41:31-57, 1994.

Henretig FM, Shannon M: Toxicologic emergencies. In Fleisher GR, Ludwig S, eds: *Textbook of pediatric emergency medicine*, ed 3, Baltimore, 1993, Williams & Wilkins, pp 745-799.

Sugarman JM, Paul RI: Flumazenil: a review, *Pediatr Emerg Care* 10:37-43, 1994.

CIRCULATION
11. Shock—Sepsis
STEPHEN J. TEACH

OBJECTIVES
1. Recognize the presentation of septic shock.
2. Manage relative hypovolemia.
3. Recognize and manage acidosis, hypoglycemia, and respiratory insufficiency.

Brief Presenting History

One-month-old infant in father's arms with a chief complaint of lethargy and poor feeding.

Initial Vital Signs

P 200, BP 50/20, RR 60.
If asked: T 38.1° C, estimated weight 4 kg.

Initial Physical Examination

General appearance: Pale, gray, mottled, limp.
If asked: Eyes closed, minimally responsive to painful stimuli.
- **Airway:** Patent.
- **Breathing:** Breath sounds full and clear symmetrically without wheezing.
- **Circulation:** Heart tones remarkable for tachycardia only. Capillary refill time 4 to 5 seconds, pulses weak.
- Pupils equal and reactive, anterior fontanel flat, no retinal hemorrhages.
- Abdomen nondistended, bowel sounds hypoactive, soft without mass.
- Rectal tone normal, stool heme negative.
- No external signs of trauma.

Further History Given on Request

Child failed to wake for feeding as expected. Parents unable to arouse him. Refuses to take the breast. No history of ingestion or trauma. Exclusively breast fed. No urine output for more than 12 hours.
- Full term, normal spontaneous vaginal delivery, uncomplicated pregnancy, labor, and delivery.
- No medications.

Expected interventions	Complications
1. 100% oxygen by face mask (proper fit).	Vomits, requiring suction.
2. Monitors (ECG and pulse oximeter).	
3. IV access attempts.	Unable to start IV, necessitating IO placement.
Continue IV attempts after IO placement.	
Consider femoral CVL.	
4. **Normal saline** 20 ml/kg IO bolus.	
5. Laboratory tests: Rapid glucose, ABG, CBC, blood culture, electrolytes, glucose, UA/UC.	
6. Antibiotics: **Ceftriaxone** 100 mg/kg IO and **ampicillin** 100 mg/kg IO.	

Initial Laboratory Findings

Rapid glucose 20, ABG: pH 7.02, P_{CO_2} 45, P_{O_2} 160.

Repeat Vital Signs

P 60, BP not obtainable, RR 10. ECG monitor shows bradycardia only. Pulse oximeter is not functioning.

Progression

Mottled color becoming blue, agonal respirations, no response to needle sticks.

Expected interventions	Complications
1. Bag-valve-mask with 100% O_2.	
2. Rapid sequence intubation.	Unable to visualize cords secondary to secretions, necessitating suctioning.
No. 1.0 Miller blade, 4.0 ETT.	Light goes out, requiring BVM.
Atropine 0.02 mg/kg IO/IV, minimum dose 0.1 mg.	Profound bradycardia if less than minimum dose of **atropine** used.
Cricoid pressure.	Vomits if no cricoid pressure applied.
Place NG and end-tidal CO_2 monitor.	Right mainstem intubation.
Call for CXR for ETT position.	Tube falls out if not taped properly.
3. Second 20 ml/kg **normal saline**, followed by **5% albumin** 20 ml/kg IV/IO.	
4. $D_{10}W$ infusion 10 ml/kg IV/IO or $D_{25}W$ 4 ml/kg IV/IO (1 g/kg).	

Progression

During intubation monitor reads asystole.

Expected interventions	Complications
1. Check pulses and ECG leads.	Pulseless.
2. Begin chest compressions.	
3. **Epinephrine** 1:10,000, 0.1 ml/kg IO/IV, or **epinephrine** 1:1000, 0.1 ml/kg ETT.	
4. Consider sodium bicarbonate 1 mEq/kg IO/IV.	Sodium bicarbonate must *not* be given via the ETT.

◆

Repeat Vital Signs

After above resuscitation: P 190, BP 75/35, perfusion improved slightly.

Potential Complications

1. Hypotension refractory to fluid management. Consider inotropic support starting with **dopamine** at 10 μg/kg/min continuous IV infusion.
2. Seizure caused by hypoxia, hypoglycemia, acidosis, or meningeal irritation initially requiring **lorazepam** 0.1 mg/kg IV, followed by **phenobarbital** 10 to 20 mg/kg IV, and if needed **paraldehyde** 7 ml/kg in glass syringe PR for seizures refractory to benzodiazepine and barbiturates. (Paraldehyde is no longer available in many hospital pharmacies.) Consider empiric **pyridoxine** 100 mg IV for infants without a seizure history.
3. Coagulopathy caused by disseminated intravascular coagulation, requiring fresh frozen plasma.
4. Pneumothorax caused by overzealous bag ventilations, necessitating thoracentesis and chest tube placement.

Disposition

ICU for ongoing management of septic shock and metabolic abnormalities.

Discussion of Objectives

1. *Recognize the presentation of septic shock.*
   Septic shock is a syndrome of inadequate end organ perfusion requiring oxygen, intravascular fluid resuscitation, and antibiotics. Symptoms of shock evident in this patient include history of decreased activity, poor oral intake, and decreased urine output. Signs of shock are tachycardia, poor perfusion with cyanosis, prolonged capillary refill time and mottled skin, and altered mental status. Hypotension as displayed by low blood pressure is a *late* finding of shock in pediatrics and is indicative of impending cardiovascular collapse.
2. *Manage relative hypovolemia.*
   Isotonic crystalloid solution is administered initially as an IV bolus, 20 ml/kg, over a short period (<15 minutes). If reassessment of the patient's condition reveals persistent poor perfusion, the 20 ml/kg bolus is repeated and then followed by colloid (i.e., **5% albumin** as a 20 ml/kg bolus). Patients with shock refractory to fluid resuscitation require inotropic support in the form of a continuous IV infusion of **dopamine** 10 to 20 μg/kg/min or **epinephrine** 0.1 to 1 μg/kg/min.

3. *Recognize and manage acidosis, hypoglycemia, and respiratory insufficiency.*
   Glucose should be administered either as $D_{10}W$ at 5 to 10 ml/kg or $D_{25}W$ at 2 to 4 ml/kg to deliver **dextrose**, approximately 0.5 to 1 g/kg.
   Use of **sodium bicarbonate** is controversial. It is typically used only in cases of severe metabolic acidosis (pH <7.20) when cardiovascular stability is compromised and when effective ventilation has reversed the respiratory component of the acidosis.
   Dosage of $NaHCO_3$ is 0.5 to 1 mEq/kg IV.

REFERENCES

Jafari HS, McCracken GH: Sepsis and septic shock: a review for clinicians, *Pediatr Infect Dis J* 11:739-749, 1992.

Saez-Llorens X, McCracken GH: Sepsis syndrome and septic shock in pediatrics: current concepts of terminology, pathophysiology, and management, *J Pediatr* 123:497-508, 1993.

12. Shock—Meningococcemia

ANNE M. STACK

OBJECTIVES

1. Recognize the syndrome of fever and petechiae as a medical emergency.
2. Understand that systolic blood pressure can be preserved late into the course of shock in children.
3. Know that early and aggressive fluid resuscitation and vasopressor therapy are lifesaving.

Brief Presenting History

A 16-month-old child awakes from his afternoon nap with fever, fussiness, and lethargy. He is pale, refuses to drink, and looks bad to his mother, who brings him in for evaluation.

Initial Vital Signs

HR 190, RR 36 (grunting), BP 87/33.
If asked: T 38.8° C, pulse oximetry 98% (room air), estimated weight 12 kg.

Physical Examination on Arrival

General appearance: Pale, lethargic, tachypneic, grunting, mottled with cool extremities.
If asked: Fine pinpoint petechiae on chest, abdomen, face.
- **Airway:** Patent.
- **Breathing:** Grunting respirations, lungs clear.
- **Circulation:** Tachycardic with regular rhythm, capillary refill time 4 to 5 seconds.
- HEENT normal.
- Abdomen soft.
- Neurologic: Lethargic, responds only to vigorous shaking and painful stimuli.

Further History Given on Request

The patient appeared well to his mother in the morning, except maybe a little less playful than usual. She noticed a fine rash on his face and chest on arrival at the hospital. The mother runs a small unlicensed day care center in her own home. The patient has a history of recurrent ear infections.
- No medications, NKDA.
- Parents do not believe in immunizations, so the child has received none.

Expected interventions	Complications
1. 100% O_2 by face mask with nonrebreather.	Vomits, requiring suction.
2. Monitors (ECG, oximeter).	
3. Attempt IV access.	Unable to start IV, necessitating IO placement.
4. Laboratory tests: Rapid glucose, ABG, CBC, blood culture, PT/PTT, fibrinogen, fibrin split products, clot to blood bank, electrolytes, AST, ALT.	
5. **Normal saline** or **Ringer's lactate** 20 ml/kg IV/IO.	
6. **Ceftriaxone** 100 mg/kg IV/IO.	
7. Place Foley catheter, send for UA/UC.	
8. Attempt central IV access (femoral).	

Progression

Rapid glucose 20 to 40, capillary refill 4 to 5 seconds.

Expected interventions	Complications
1. **$D_{25}W$** 2 to 4 ml/kg IV push (0.5 to 1 g/kg).	$D_{25}W$ infiltrates peripheral line.
2. Repeat **NS** 20 ml/kg IV bolus. Infuse through IO or CVL.	

Initial Laboratory Findings

ABG: pH 7.18, P_{CO_2} 35, P_{O_2} 145, base excess −9.

Repeat Vital Signs

After first 20 ml/kg of normal saline: HR 188, BP 86/32, RR 18.

Progression

Respirations slow. Increasing grunting with pulse oximeter at 91%. Rash is evolving to purpuric in nature over entire body.

Expected interventions	Complications
1. Rapid sequence intubation. No. 2.0 Miller blade, 4.5 ETT. **Atropine** 0.02 mg/kg IV/IO. **Midazolam** 0.1 mg/kg IV/IO. **Vecuronium** 0.1 to 0.2 mg/kg IV/IO. Cricoid pressure. Place NG and end-tidal CO_2 monitor. Call for CXR to check ETT position. 2. Consider **albumin** or **FFP** 20 ml/kg IV. 3. Begin **dopamine** at 10 μg/kg/min continuous IV infusion. 4. Notify ICU physicians. 5. Recheck rapid glucose.	Ambu bag will not inflate, not plugged into flow meter. Vomiting because cricoid pressure released too soon, necessitating suction. ETT falls out because of poor tape job, necessitating BVM and reintubation.

Laboratory Results

Rapid glucose 50, WBC 1.3 (88P 10B 2L), Hct 33%, Plts 101K, Na 139, K 4.6, Cl 107, CO_2 8, ionized calcium 0.8 mmol/L, PT 14, PTT 41, fibrinogen 123, fibrin split products >100.

Expected interventions	Complications
1. $D_{25}W$ 2 to 4 ml/kg IV push (0.5 to 1 g/kg). 2. Give 10% $CaCl_2$ 0.2 ml/kg slow IV push. 3. Consider **heparin** 50 U/kg bolus followed by 25 U/kg/hr continuous IV infusion.	Failure to treat hypoglycemia leads to seizure. $CaCl_2$ given too fast leads to bradycardia, necessitating **atropine** 0.02 mg/kg IV.

Additional Potential Complications

1. Rapid glucose is not checked. Patient has a generalized seizure refractory to **lorazepam** 0.1 mg/kg.
2. Insufficient fluid resuscitation leads to a precipitous fall in blood pressure; the patient then has a full cardiopulmonary arrest, necessitating CPR and IV **epinephrine** 1:1000, 0.1 ml/kg IV.
3. During unnecessary lumbar puncture attempt, the patient has a full cardiorespiratory arrest, necessitating CPR.
4. Caretakers fail to wear masks and require **rifampin** prophylaxis.

Disposition

ICU.

Discussion of Objectives

1. *Recognize the syndrome of fever and petechiae as a medical emergency.*
   Fever and petechiae may be signs of overwhelming bacterial infection and must be treated as a true medical emergency. Caretakers must observe strict respiratory precautions. The patient requires emergency triage. Antibiotics must be given by IV push immediately after a blood culture is obtained. *Do not* delay administration of antibiotics for obtaining urine or CSF culture. Immediate intervention may be lifesaving or limb saving.

2. *Understand that systolic blood pressure can be preserved late into the course of shock in children.*
   Because in children the heart can massively increase output by increasing heart rate (rather than stroke volume), blood pressure is preserved until relatively late. Tachycardia is a much earlier indicator of relative hypovolemic shock in pediatric patients. However, tachycardia is a nonspecific indicator that may be present in patients with fever, pain, or distress from visiting the doctor. Tachycardia must be addressed further through checking other indicators of hypovolemia, such as skin color, temperature, and turgor, capillary refill time, and quality of peripheral pulses. A wide pulse pressure, indicative of low systemic vascular resistance resulting from the endotoxin effect of endogenous inflammatory mediators, may be a clue that shock is imminent.

3. *Know that early and aggressive fluid resuscitation and vasopressor therapy are lifesaving.*
   Low systemic vascular resistance is an indication that the patient is experiencing distributive shock. Fluid as isotonic crystalloid must be given aggressively, initially at 20 to 40 ml/kg, to prevent the sequelae of hypoperfusion and shock.
   Endotoxin leads to release of myocardial depressant factor. Administration of vasopressors with beta agonist activity improves inotropy and subsequently cardiac output. Vasopressors can also improve vascular tone and increase systemic vascular resistance.
   The use of colloid should be considered early, certainly after 20 ml/kg boluses of saline have been given twice. In a patient with disseminated intravascular coagulation, fresh frozen plasma is the colloid of choice to replenish clotting factors.

Additional Comments

1. There is no evidence that high-dose steroid therapy is efficacious in meningococcemia, and some data suggest that steroids in high doses (30 mg/kg) may be harmful. If adrenal infarction (Waterhouse-Friderichsen syndrome) is suspected, "stress dose" steroids (**methylprednisolone** 2 mg/kg) should be considered.

2. **Thiopental** should not be used for intubation in this situation because its peripheral vasodilatory effects may exacerbate hypotension.

3. The use of **heparin** in purpura fulminans (meningococcemia) is controversial, although some authors support its use to prevent the clotting sequelae that may lead to loss of digits or limbs.

4. The use of **calcium chloride (CaCl$_2$)** in this scenario is in response to hypocalcemia as documented by an ionized calcium of 0.8. The role of calcium in pediatric resuscitation has changed. Its use is now indicated only in documented hypocalcemia, hyperkalemia, hypermagnesemia, or

in calcium channel blocker ingestions or toxicity. The pediatric dose is 0.2 ml/kg (20 mg/kg of the salt and 5.4 mg/kg of elemental calcium) 10% (100 mg/ml) **calcium chloride** solution by *slow* IV push. The adult dose is $CaCl_2$ 2 to 10 ml (0.2 to 1 g) *slow* IV push.

Note: Rapid infusion of calcium solutions results in bradycardia.

REFERENCES

Bell LM, Fleisher GR: Shock and infectious diseases emergencies. In Fleisher GR, Ludwig S, eds: *Textbook of pediatric emergency medicine*, ed 3, Baltimore, 1993, Williams & Wilkins, pp 44-54, 596-600.

Bone KC et al: A controlled trial of high dose methylprednisolone in the treatment of severe sepsis and septic shock, *N Engl J Med* 317:653-658, 1987.

Carcillo JA, Davis AL, Zaritsky A: Role of early fluid resuscitation in pediatric septic shock, *JAMA* 266:1242-1245, 1991.

Malley R, Huskins C, Kuppermann N: Multivariable predictive models for adverse outcome of invasive meningococcal disease in children, *J Pediatr* 129:702-710, 1996.

13. Shock—Gastrointestinal Bleeding—Iron Ingestion

STEPHEN J. TEACH

OBJECTIVES
1. Recognize the presentation of hypovolemic shock.
2. Manage gastrointestinal hemorrhage and hypovolemia.
3. Manage the complications of iron ingestion.

Brief Presenting History

A 2-year-old arrives in his grandmother's arms with a chief complaint of bloody vomitus and lethargy.

Initial Vital Signs

P 164, BP 75/30, RR 40.
If asked: T 38.2° C (R). Estimated weight 13 kg.

Initial Physical Examination

General appearance: Pale, ill-appearing, lethargic toddler with bloody vomitus dripping from his nose.
If asked: Eyes open, awake, poorly responsive.
- **Airway:** Patent.
- **Breathing:** Breath sounds symmetric and clear.
- **Circulation:** Heart tones significant for tachycardia only. Capillary refill time 3 to 4 seconds.
- Pupils 4 mm, symmetric and reactive, anicteric.
- No signs of external trauma.
- Abdomen distended, diffusely tender in epigastrium.
- Bright red blood per rectum, tone normal, strongly heme positive.

Further History Given on Request

The child was being watched by his grandmother, who found him in a pool of bloody emesis. An empty pill bottle was found under the kitchen table. The grandmother did not bring the bottle but says they were for "low blood counts."
- Previous medical history unremarkable.
- NKDA.
- No medications.
- Fully immunized.

Expected interventions	Complications
1. 100% oxygen, BVM-assisted breaths as needed. Prepare for rapid sequence intubation.	
2. Monitors (ECG, oximeter).	
3. IV access attempts.	If unable to start peripheral IV, place IO and attempt femoral CVL.
4. **Normal saline** 20 ml/kg IV.	
5. Consider call to blood bank for **O-negative blood**.	
6. Laboratory tests: Rapid glucose, ABG, CBC, type and cross, electrolytes, liver function tests, iron/TIBC, toxicologic screen.	
7. NG versus larger bore OG to evacuate stomach contents.	
8. Flat plate film of the abdomen.	

Initial Laboratory Findings

Rapid glucose 120, ABG: pH 7.18, P_{CO_2} 30, P_{O_2} 280.

Repeat Vital Signs

P 180, BP not obtainable, RR 25, pulse oximeter not functioning.

Progression

Increasing somnolence, unresponsive to painful stimulation, respiratory effort minimal.

Expected interventions	Complications
1. BVM-assisted breaths with 100% oxygen.	Vomiting if no cricoid pressure applied.
2. Rapid sequence intubation.	Unable to visualize cords secondary to secretions requiring suctioning.
No. 2.0 Mac/Miller blade.	Laryngoscope light not functioning.
4.5 ETT.	Copious hematemesis.
Atropine 0.02 mg/kg IV.	Right mainstem intubation.
Midazolam 0.1 mg/kg IV.	Vomits if no cricoid pressure is applied or NG not placed.
Rocuronium 0.6 to 1 mg/kg IV or **vecuronium** 0.1 to 0.2 mg/kg IV.	Tube falls out if not properly taped and attended.
Cricoid pressure.	
Place NG and end-tidal CO_2 monitor.	
CXR for ETT position.	
3. Continue volume resuscitation.	
Repeat 20 ml/kg **normal saline** followed by 20 ml/kg **5% albumin**.	
Consider unmatched **O-negative blood**.	
4. Consider **sodium bicarbonate** 1 mEq/kg IV.	

Repeat Vital Signs

P 150, BP 90/60, perfusion improved.

Laboratory Tests

Glucose 180, Hct 34, WBC 25,000, ABG: pH 7.20, P_{CO_2} 30, P_{O_2} 220.
Flat plate film of abdomen: radiopaque objects in stomach and small bowel.

Expected Interventions

1. Gastric lavage using 2% to 5% **sodium bicarbonate solution**.
2. **Deferoxamine** 15 mg/kg/hr continuous IV infusion ASAP.
3. Repeat abdominal flat plate film after gastric lavage.

Additional Potential Complications

1. Bradycardia and arrest caused by hypoxia or acidosis if airway is not secured.
2. Seizure caused by hypoxia or acidosis requiring **lorazepam** 0.1 mg/kg IV, followed by **phenytoin** 10 to 20 mg/kg IV load over 20 minutes. (If phenytoin given too fast, cardiovascular collapse occurs.)
3. Coagulopathy caused by hepatic toxicity requiring **fresh frozen plasma**.
4. Potential exists for acute onset of coma, shock, seizures, sepsis, and profound hepatic toxicity and failure.

Disposition

ICU for further bowel decontamination and ongoing management of hemorrhagic shock, iron chelation, and hepatic toxicity.

Discussion of Objectives

1. *Recognize the presentation of hemorrhagic shock.*
   Shock is a syndrome of inadequate end organ perfusion requiring oxygen and aggressive intravascular fluid resuscitation. This patient has tachycardia and poor skin perfusion, which are initial signs of shock in pediatric patients, but also displays later signs such as compromised blood pressure and altered mental status.
2. *Manage GI hemorrhage and hypovolemia.*
   Hypovolemic shock in pediatric patients is treated initially with isotonic crystalloid at 20 ml/kg by rapid IV bolus. If reassessment reveals ongoing compromised perfusion, the 20 ml/kg bolus is repeated. Persistent hypovolemia despite isotonic crystalloid 40 ml/kg is treated with 20 ml/kg IV of colloid such as 5% albumin. Patients refractory to this aggressive therapy should be considered for unmatched O-negative blood in an acute situation followed by cross-matched blood as time allows. Close attention should be paid to ongoing losses. Reassess perfusion after each fluid bolus.
3. *Manage the complications of iron ingestion.*
   Ingested iron acts directly on the mucosa of the GI tract, leading to hemorrhagic necrosis of the stomach and intestines. Liver injury is secondary to the presence of free iron in the circulation.

Rapid gut decontamination is a high priority. This is accomplished by gastric lavage followed by whole bowel irrigation and endoscopy if repeat abdominal films reveal persistent iron pill fragments or a bezoar.

In severe ingestions serum iron chelation is accomplished using IV **deferoxamine** 15 mg/kg/hr. Parenteral deferoxamine therapy enhances the excretion of iron. If the amount of iron ingested is in doubt and serum iron measurements are not readily available, a deferoxamine challenge may be given. **Deferoxamine** 50 mg/kg (up to 1 g) IM is administered, and a pinkish orange urine indicates the presence of iron-deferoxamine complex. When this complex is present, significant serum iron levels may be expected and chelation therapy undertaken.

Additional Comments

1. In the management of metabolic acidosis the use of **sodium bicarbonate** is controversial and should be reserved for severe acidosis (pH <7.20) when accompanied by cardiovascular instability. Patients receiving sodium bicarbonate therapy must have the ability to excrete the products of bicarbonate metabolism, most importantly carbon dioxide.
2. Gastric lavage is performed with **2% to 5% sodium bicarbonate** solution to convert free ferrous salts to insoluble ferrous carbonate, which decreases both absorption and corrosive effects.
   a. Activated charcoal does not absorb iron and is not recommended unless ingestion of other agents is suspected.
   b. Whole bowel irrigation has a potential role but should be used cautiously in patients with active GI bleeding or ileus.
3. Severe iron intoxication produces leukocytosis, hyperglycemia, metabolic acidosis, and liver injury evidenced by hyperbilirubinemia, increased liver enzyme levels, and a prolonged prothrombin time.

REFERENCES

Lacouture PG et al: Emergency assessment of severity in iron overdose by clinical and laboratory methods, *J Pediatr* 99:89, 1981.
McGuigan MA: Acute iron poisoning, *Pediatr Ann* 25:33-38, 1996.
Woo OF: Iron. In Olson KR, ed: *Poisoning and drug overdose*, Norwalk, Conn, 1990, Appleton & Lange, pp 63-65.

14. Shock—Cardiogenic—Myocarditis

RICHARD BACHUR

OBJECTIVES
1. Recognize respiratory failure.
2. Recognize and manage cardiogenic shock.
3. Manage ventricular tachycardia without a pulse.
4. Treat cardiogenic shock.

Brief Presenting History

A 4-year-old girl is brought in with respiratory distress. She was seen by her doctor 2 days ago, noted to have significant wheezing, and begun on home nebulizer therapy and steroids. Over the 2 days she has experienced increasingly more labored breathing and listlessness.

Initial Vital Signs

P 150, BP 100/85, RR 36, estimated weight 15 kg.

Initial Physical Examination

General appearance: Anxious little girl, sitting up, in moderate respiratory distress, sleepy, but answers questions appropriately. Circumoral cyanosis present.
If asked:
- **Airway:** Patent, patient speaks.
- **Breathing:** Moderate intercostal and subcostal retractions are present. Diffuse expiratory wheezing, crackles present throughout lung fields.
- **Circulation:** Heart tones difficult to hear because of respiratory noise, thready peripheral pulses. Cool, slightly mottled extremities, capillary refill time 3 to 4 seconds.
- Jugular venous distention (JVD) present during exhalation.
- Liver edge palpated 3 cm below right costal margin.

Further History if Requested

Recent URI but now no fever or runny nose. No ill contacts.
- Unremarkable past medical history. No medications before 3 days ago.
- NKDA, family history negative for asthma.

Expected interventions	Complications
1. Apply oxygen.	Initially refuses to lie down.
2. Monitors (ECG, oximeter).	
3. IV access attempts.	Agitation with IV attempts, which are
4. Call for CXR.	unsuccessful.
5. ABG.	No response to nebulizer if given.

Progression

Somnolent between IV attempts, slowing respirations, becomes apneic.

Expected interventions	Complications
1. BVM with 100% O_2.	Vomits if no cricoid pressure applied.
2. Place IO needle.	First IO attempt infiltrates.
Hang **normal saline**.	If fluid bolus given, respiratory distress worsens.
3. Prepare for rapid sequence intubation.	

Progression

Monitor reads ventricular tachycardia. (See p. 219 in Appendix E.)

Expected interventions	Complications
1. Check pulses.	No pulses palpable.
2. Begin chest compressions.	
Assess by palpating femoral pulse.	
3. Continue BVM with 100% O_2.	
4. **Defibrillate** 2 joules/kg asynchronous mode.	
5. Reassess.	

Progression

Monitor shows sinus rhythm, rate 180. Patient is unconscious.

Laboratory Findings

Rapid glucose 120, ABG: pH 7.05, Pco_2 50, Po_2 85, HCO_3 14.

Expected interventions	Complications
1. Check pulses.	Pulses present.
2. Rapid sequence intubation.	Vomits if no cricoid pressure applied.
BVM, 100% O_2, suction.	
5.0 ETT, Miller no. 2 blade.	
Atropine 0.02 mg/kg IV/IO.	
+/−**Midazolam** 0.1 mg/kg IV/IO.	If no sedation or paralytics, patient awakes
+/−**Vecuronium** 0.1 to 0.2 mg/kg IV/IO.	and pulls out ETT.
Cricoid pressure.	
Place NG and end-tidal CO_2 monitor.	Right mainstem intubation.
Call for CXR to check ETT position.	Vomits and becomes difficult to bag if no
	NG placed.
3. Attempt further IV access, attempt CVL.	

Progression

Monitor shows ventricular tachycardia. (See p. 219 in Appendix E.)

Expected interventions	Complications
1. Check pulses.	No pulse palpated.
2. Chest compressions.	Monitor shows ventricular fibrillation or
Defibrillate 2 joules/kg asynchronous.	tachycardia.
3. Check pulses.	No pulse palpated.
4. Chest compressions.	Monitor shows ventricular fibrillation or
Defibrillate 2 joules/kg asynchronous.	tachycardia.
5. **Lidocaine** 1 mg/kg IV/IO bolus.	
6. Check pulses.	Still no pulse.
7. Chest compressions.	
Defibrillate 4 joules/kg asynchronous.	

Progression

Femoral pulses now palpable, crackles and wheezes throughout lung fields, heart tones significant for obvious gallop. CXR reveals large cardiac silhouette and pulmonary edema.

Expected interventions

1. Inotrope, **dobutamine** 10 to 20 μg/kg/min continuous IV infusion.
2. Consider **lidocaine** 25 μg/kg/min continuous IV infusion after bolus is given.
3. Positive end-expiratory pressure (PEEP) with ventilation.
4. **Furosemide** 1 mg/kg IV.
5. Obtain additional IV access—femoral CVL.
6. Place Foley catheter.

7. ECG.
8. Consult cardiology department.

Potential Complications

1. Aggressive positive-pressure ventilation before or after intubation leads to pneumothorax requiring needle thoracostomy and chest tube placement.
2. Defibrillator ineffective if used in synchronous mode.

Disposition

ICU.

Discussion of Objectives

1. *Recognize respiratory failure.*
   The criteria for respiratory failure are highly variable. The major clinical parameters are severe respiratory distress with significantly increased work of breathing, including massive accessory respiratory muscle usage and severe retractions followed by poor respiratory effort or agonal breathing. This leads to decreased or absent breath sounds, cyanosis, decreased level of consciousness, and finally apnea. Strict physiologic criteria include $Paco_2$ >40 with severe distress (evidence of CO_2 retention), and Pao_2 <60 on 40% inspired oxygen.

2. *Recognize and manage cardiogenic shock.*
   In addition to the usual features of the clinical presentation of shock, cardiogenic shock may have the following features: distended neck veins, congested lungs with crackles or wheezes on auscultation, hepatomegaly, gallop rhythm, and muffled heart tones (pericardial tamponade).
   Other clues to the diagnosis of cardiogenic shock include paradoxic response to fluid challenge, large cardiac silhouette on radiograph, narrow pulse pressure, low mixed venous Po_2, and ECG changes (specifically decreased magnitude of forces and ST-T wave changes consistent with myocardial or pericardial disease).
   Cardiogenic shock can be due to dysrhythmias, drug intoxication, hypoxia, ischemia, acidosis, hypothermia, hypoglycemia, myopathies, or pericardial disease (restrictive or tamponade).
   Common scenarios for cardiogenic shock are infants with shock during the first few weeks of life (caused by ductal-dependent lesions such as hypoplastic left heart, coarctation of the aorta or aortic stenosis, and anomalous left coronary artery; see mock code 7, Respiratory Distress—Coarctation of the Aorta, p. 44), older infants with large left-to-right shunts who have congestive heart failure, and atypical courses for wheezing and pneumonia that actually represent myocarditis.

3. *Manage ventricular tachycardia without a pulse.*
   Ventricular tachycardia without a pulse is treated the same as ventricular fibrillation. The algorithm consists of securing an airway and initiating CPR, then **defibrillation** at 2 joules/kg in the asynchronous mode. For persistent ventricular tachycardia without a pulse or ventricular fibrillation, defibrillation should be repeated at 4 joules/kg. This may be repeated a third time if the initial two attempts are unsuccessful.
   If no response, **epinephrine** can be given (ET/IO/IV) with repeat **defibrillation** after 60 seconds. If still no response, additional **epinephrine** can be given every 3 minutes, along with a

bolus of **lidocaine** (followed by defibrillation). If defibrillation is still unsuccessful, give **bretylium** 5 mg/kg followed by defibrillation within 30 to 60 seconds. If no response, repeat **bretylium** 10 mg/kg followed by defibrillation within 30 to 60 seconds.

Correction of acidosis and other metabolic abnormalities must also be considered. The defibrillation dosage recommendations for adults are 200-300-360 joules.

See Tachycardia (p. 200) in Chapter 4.

4. *Treat cardiogenic shock.*

Once recognized, the treatment for a poor functioning myocardium consists of:

a. Ensuring adequate preload but not overloading with fluids.

b. Inotropic support (preferentially without increasing the systemic vascular resistance [SVR]; i.e., best to use dobutamine, dopamine, or amrinone rather than epinephrine or norepinephrine).

c. Diuresis once inotropic support begins and adequate blood pressure and perfusion are restored.

Management is greatly facilitated with a CVP monitor or Swan-Ganz catheter. Once inotropic support is begun, afterload reduction may also be beneficial. If the cardiogenic shock is based on pericardial fluid, maximizing preload and inotropic support is indicated while preparing for pericardiocentesis.

Advance management centers on monitoring blood pressure, mental status, urine output, acidosis, oxygenation, and CVP (or preferably with pulmonary artery wedge pressures and cardiac outputs).

REFERENCES

Bonadio WA, Losek JD: Infants with myocarditis presenting with severe respiratory distress and shock, *Pediatr Emerg Care* 3:110-113, 1987.

Flynn PA, Engle MA, Ehlers KH: Cardiac issues in the pediatric emergency room, *Pediatr Clin North Am* 39:955-995, 1992.

Hohn AR, Stanton RE: Myocarditis in children, *Pediatr Rev* 9:83-88, 1987.

Press S, Lipkind RS: Acute myocarditis in infants, *Clin Pediatr* 29:73-76, 1990.

15. Shock—Congenital Adrenal Hyperplasia

LEWIS R. FIRST

OBJECTIVES

1. Recognize and manage seizures secondary to hyponatremia and/or hypoglycemia.
2. Manage asystole.
3. Recognize and manage the complications of congenital adrenal hyperplasia.

Brief Presenting History

Three-week-old male infant found having a seizure in his crib.

Initial Vital Signs

HR 180, BP 30/P, RR 80.
If asked: T 38° C (R), estimated weight 4 kg.

Initial Physical Examination

General appearance: Generalized tonic-clonic seizure.
If asked: Circumoral and peripheral cyanosis.
- **Airway:** Patent.
- **Breathing:** Tachypneic, lungs clear.
- **Circulation:** Weak pulses with normal heart sounds, capillary refill time 5 seconds.
- Over 10% dehydrated (decreased skin turgor, sunken fontanel).
- Pupils equal, dilated, sluggishly reactive.
- Abdomen soft, nondistended.
- Scrotum hyperpigmented.

Further History Given on Request

Full-term, normal spontaneous vaginal delivery, home on day 2 of life. Past 3 days with decreased oral intake. Vomiting and diarrhea over last 2 days, decreased number of wet diapers. Poor breast-feeding and failure to take bottle supplements yesterday.

Expected interventions	Complications

1. 100% O_2 by face mask.
2. Monitors (ECG and pulse oximeter).
3. Attempt IV access.
    Normal saline 20 ml/kg IV/IO.
    Laboratory tests: Rapid glucose, ABG,
        electrolytes, CBC, blood culture.
4. **Lorazepam** 0.05 to 0.1 mg/kg IV/IO or
    diazepam 0.5 mg/kg PR.
	Unsuccessful IV attempt, requiring IO placement.

Laboratory Results

Rapid glucose <20, ABG: pH 7.01, P_{CO_2} 28, P_{O_2}, 45, Na 124, K 7.2, Cl 97, HCO_3 4.

Progression

Seizure stops, but patient vomits and aspirates.

Expected interventions	Complications
1. Suction, clear airway. 2. **$D_{10}W$** 5 to 10 ml/kg IV/IO or **$D_{25}W$** 2 to 4 ml/kg IV/IO.	Vomiting.

Progression

Blood pressure unobtainable, patient stops breathing, asystole develops.

Expected interventions	Complications
1. Bag-valve-mask with 100% O_2.	Improper depth and rate of respirations and compressions.
Cricoid pressure.	Vomits if no cricoid pressure applied.

2. Initiate chest compressions.
3. Rapid sequence intubation.
    Miller no. 0 blade, 3.5 ETT.
    Place NG and end-tidal CO_2 monitor.
    Call for CXR for ETT position.
	Light of laryngoscope out.
	Copious secretions requiring suction.

4. **Epinephrine** 1:10,000, 0.1 ml/kg IV/IO. 5. **Epinephrine** 1:1000, 0.1 ml/kg IV/IO.	Persistent asystole.

Progression

Monitor reads sinus rhythm, rate of 160.

Expected interventions	Progression and complications
1. Check pulses.	Pulse present.
2. Repeat **normal saline** 20 ml/kg IV/IO.	IV infiltrates.

Progression

Pulseless ventricular tachycardia or ventricular fibrillation develops.

Expected interventions	Progression and complications
1. Chest compressions.	
2. **Defibrillate:** Asynchronous mode, 2 joules/kg.	Sinus rhythm 170.
3. Treat hyperkalemia.	
10% calcium gluconate 30 mg/kg IV or	
10% CaCl$_2$ 0.2 ml/kg slow IVP.	
Sodium bicarbonate 1 mEq/kg IV.	
Hyperventilate.	
Consider **glucose** 1 g/kg IV and **insulin** 1 unit	Incorrect doses lead to hypoglycemia
per 5 g glucose.	and seizure.
Consider **albuterol** 2.5 mg nebulizer.	
4. When stable, 12-lead ECG.	
5. Once the acute adrenal crisis caused by congenital adrenal hyperplasia is recognized, give a bolus of **hydrocortisone** 25 mg IV or **deoxycorticosterone acetate** (DOCA) 1 mg IM.	

Additional Potential Complications

1. Persistent hypotension may require inotropic support.
2. Hyperkalemia may result in idioventricular rhythms or ventricular fibrillation, as well as asystole described above.

Disposition

ICU.

Discussion of Objectives

1. *Recognize and manage seizures caused by hyponatremia or hypoglycemia.*
   See mock code 19, Seizure—Hyponatremia, p. 96, and mock code 20, Seizure—Hypoglycemia, p. 102.

2. *Manage asystole.*

   See Asystole (p. 198) in Chapter 4.

3. *Recognize and manage the complications of congenital adrenal hyperplasia.*

   Management of acute salt wasting crisis should include the following:

   a. Dehydration. Volume expansion with rapid infusion of isotonic solution. Normal saline 20 ml/kg in the first 15 to 30 minutes. Reassess and repeat as indicated.

   b. Hypoglycemia. Initial glucose replacement with $D_{10}W$ 5 to 10 ml/kg or $D_{25}W$ 2 to 4 ml/kg (0.5 to 1 g/kg) followed by addition of D_{10} to maintenance IV fluid solution.

   c. Hyponatremia and hyperkalemia. Correction of both begins with infusion of normal saline. In the presence of seizures, hyponatremia may be treated more rapidly using **3% NaCl** 10 to 12 ml/kg, given IV over 1 hour with the goal of increasing the sodium by 10 mEq/L. Rapid infusion of 3% NaCl may result in the osmotic demyelination syndrome. Reported in adults, this potentially fatal complication of increasing the serum sodium too rapidly is seen more frequently in patients with chronic hyponatremia who are treated aggressively. (See mock code 19, Seizure—Hyponatremia, p. 96.)

   In the setting of dysrhythmias, hyperkalemia is treated with **calcium** to help stabilize myocardial cell membranes. Movement of potassium into cells is enhanced by several mechanisms, including **alkalinization**, use of a combination of **glucose** and **insulin**, and use of **albuterol**. Insulin and glucose must be used with extreme caution in this instance because hypoglycemia may result. Excretion of potassium is enhanced by administering **Kayexalate**. In extreme cases and for long-term treatment of hyperkalemia caused by renal failure, hemodialysis is used. (See mock code 24, Hyperkalemia, p. 120.) Peaked T-waves may be seen on the 12-lead ECG when significant hyperkalemia is present.

4. Steroid replacement is essential with the life-threatening entity CAH. If readily available, **deoxycorticosterone acetate (DOCA)** 1 mg IM should be given. DOCA does not interfere with the diagnostic tests that will be performed when the patient's condition stabilizes (e.g., serum 17-hydroxyprogesterone, 24-hour urinary 17-ketosteroid, and pregnenolone levels).

   Glucocorticoid replacement in the form of **hydrocortisone** 25 mg IV bolus, followed by 50 mg/mm^2/24 hr as a constant infusion, should follow. Although hydrocortisone is essential for effective treatment, its addition will suppress ACTH precursor steroid production, making the specific enzyme deficiency more difficult to diagnose.

Additional Comments

1. If a paralytic were required, **rocuronium** or **vecuronium** would be recommended. Succinylcholine would be contraindicated in this case because hyperkalemia is present.

REFERENCES

Hale DE: Endocrine emergencies. In Fleisher GR, Ludwig S, eds: *Textbook of pediatric emergency medicine*, ed 3, Baltimore, 1993, Williams & Wilkins, pp 948-950.

Saladino RA: Endocrine and metabolic disorders. In Barkin RM, ed: *Pediatric emergency medicine: concepts and clinical practice*, ed 2, St Louis, 1997, Mosby.

White PC, New MI, DuPont B: Congenital adrenal hyperplasia, *N Engl J Med* 316:1519-1524, 1987.

NEUROLOGIC PRESENTATIONS
16. Altered Mental Status—Shaken Baby Syndrome
MARK G. ROBACK

OBJECTIVES
1. Recognize the presentation of the shaken baby syndrome.
2. Manage increased intracranial pressure.
3. Manage seizures.

Brief Presenting History

A 4-month-old male is brought for treatment by his mother, who reports that he was perfectly well this morning but would not awake from his nap this afternoon.

Initial Vital Signs

P 160, BP 110/80, RR 10.
If asked: T 38° C (R), estimated weight 5 kg.

Initial Physical Examination

General appearance: Flaccid patient with mottled skin.
If asked: No cry, nonspecific movement to painful stimulus.
- **Airway:** Patent.
- **Breathing:** Agonal respirations, no crackles or wheezing.
- **Circulation:** Capillary refill time 4 seconds peripherally.
- No spontaneous eye opening, right pupil 2 mm, left pupil 4 mm, retinal hemorrhages present.
- Anterior fontanel bulging.
- Abdomen nondistended, hypoactive bowel sounds, soft.
- Extremities without bruising or obvious deformities.

Further History Given on Request

Full-term, uncomplicated pregnancy, labor, and delivery; normal spontaneous vaginal delivery. Two sets of immunizations, second set 1 week ago. Patient cared for by mother's boyfriend this afternoon.

Expected interventions	Complications
1. 100% Oxygen by face mask (proper fit).	Vomits, requiring in-line log roll and suction.
2. Immobilize cervical spine.	
3. Monitors (ECG and pulse oximeter).	
4. Attempt peripheral IV access. Continue IV attempts after IO placement. Consider femoral CVL.	Unable to start IV, necessitating IO placement.
5. **Normal saline** 20 ml/kg IV.	
6. Laboratory tests: Rapid glucose, ABG, CBC, electrolytes, BUN/Cr, LFTs, type & cross, blood culture, catheter UA/UC.	

Repeat Vital Signs

P 85, BP 60/P, RR 6.

Expected interventions	Complications
1. Bag-valve-mask ventilation with 100% O_2. Cricoid pressure.	Vomiting, if no cricoid pressure applied.
2. Prepare for rapid sequence intubation.	

Laboratory Findings

Rapid glucose 78, ABG: pH 7.02, P_{CO_2} 85, P_{O_2} 60.

Progression

Generalized tonic-clonic seizure activity.

Expected interventions	Complications
1. **Lorazepam** 0.05 to 0.1 mg/kg IV/IO.	Now apneic.
2. Rapid sequence intubation.	
Miller no. 1 blade.	
4.0 ETT.	Right mainstem intubation.
Atropine 0.02 mg/kg IV/ET, minimum dose 0.1 mg.	Bradycardia develops if less than minimum dose of atropine given.
Lidocaine 1 mg/kg IV/ET.	
Succinylcholine 1 mg/kg mg IV with defasciculating dose **vecuronium** 0.01 mg/kg IV or **vecuronium** alone 0.1 to 0.2 mg/kg IV.	Tube falls out if not properly taped and cared for.
Cricoid pressure.	
Place NG/OG and end-tidal CO_2 monitor.	No NG leads to abdominal distention and desaturation.
CXR for ETT position.	
3. Repeat normal saline 20 ml/kg IV/IO.	
4. Repeat ABG.	
5. Secondary survey: Abdomen soft, nondistended, pelvis intact, extremities with bruising but no deformities, back atraumatic, rectal heme negative.	
6. Contact neurosurgical and trauma services.	

◆

Additional Potential Complications

1. Head injuries caused by nonaccidental trauma may present a variety of signs and symptoms. Respiratory distress, seizures, asystole, and obtundation are common. Obvious signs of trauma are often absent.
2. Tense distended abdomen with further signs of hypotension leads to workup of intraabdominal trauma.

Disposition

Radiology for CT scan of head and abdomen, full skeletal survey if stable; ICU or OR depending on findings.

Discussion of Objectives

1. *Recognize the presentation of the shaken baby syndrome.*
   Impact injury from shaking must be suspected when a child, usually less than 1 year of age, is brought for treatment because of an altered level of consciousness. (See Altered Mental Status [p. 193] in Chapter 4.) Typically caregivers provide a history inconsistent with the physical findings, which may include coma, a bulging fontanel, fixed and dilated pupils, and abnormal motor posturing. In extreme cases seizures or respiratory arrest leading to asystole may occur.

Further examination may reveal retinal hemorrhages, increased head size in patients with open sutures, skeletal deformities, or bruising. However, patients may have no manifestations other than altered mental status, making the diagnosis challenging. Symptoms arise from increased intracranial pressure caused by fluid accumulation, which may occur over several days from a subdural focus, or intracerebral edema resulting from diffuse axonal injury.

Violent shaking of the infant or child, often followed by a sudden impact as the patient is thrown into a wall or against another hard surface, provides an acceleration/deceleration mechanism resulting in intracranial injury and possible injuries to the neck, chest, and extremities.

2. *Manage increased intracranial pressure.*
   See Increased Intracranial Pressure (p. 196) in Chapter 4.

3. *Manage seizures.*
   See Seizures (p. 195) in Chapter 4.

Additional Comments

See Trauma (p. 204) in Chapter 4.

REFERENCES

Bruce DA: Head trauma. Bruce DA. Neurosurgical emergencies. In Fleisher GR, Ludwig S, eds: *Textbook of pediatric emergency medicine*, ed 3, Baltimore, 1993, Williams & Wilkins, pp 1102-1112, 1410-1416.

Bruce DA, Zimmerman RA: Shaken impact syndrome, *Pediatr Ann* 18:482-494, 1989.

Duhaime AC et al: Head injury in very young children, *Pediatrics* 90:179-185, 1992.

17. Altered Mental Status—Tricyclic Antidepressant Ingestion
ERICA LIEBELT

OBJECTIVES
1. Evaluate and manage altered mental status.
2. Recognize the signs and symptoms of tricyclic antidepressant (TCA) overdose.
3. Manage the complications of TCA overdose.

Brief Presenting History

An 18-month-old female was found sleeping on the living room floor by her mother, who could not arouse her. The mother states that she was fine earlier in the day and has not been sick recently.

Initial Vital Signs

P 180, BP 120/58, RR 22.
If asked: T 37.3° C (R), estimated weight 12 kg.

Initial Physical Examination

General appearance: Comatose; no obvious signs of external injury.
If asked: Moans when vigorously stimulated; no eye opening on command.
- **Airway:** Patent.
- **Breathing:** Lungs clear, breath sounds full bilaterally.
- **Circulation:** Tachycardic, well perfused, brisk pulses.
- Pupils 4 to 5 mm and reactive.
- Skin dry and red.
- Abdomen nondistended, soft, nontender.
- Reflexes 1+, symmetric; no focal neurologic signs.

Expected interventions	*Complications*
1. 100% O_2 by face mask.	
2. Monitors (ECG and oximeter).	
3. Establish IV access.	IV access unsuccessful, necessitating IO placement. Unable to draw blood for laboratory tests.
4. Obtain blood for laboratory tests by arterial stick: Rapid glucose, ABG, CBC, electrolytes.	
5. **Naloxone** 0.1 mg/kg IV/IO.	
6. Prepare for rapid sequence intubation.	

Further History Given on Request

The child was visiting at her grandmother's house earlier in the day. Grandma has a history of depression and takes medication. The patient has a past history of lead poisoning but otherwise is healthy and takes no medications.

Laboratory Findings

Preintubation glucose 120, ABG: pH 7.32, P_{CO_2} 47, P_{O_2} 126, base deficit −6.

Progression

Generalized tonic-clonic seizure.

Expected interventions	Complications
1. **Lorazepam** 0.05 to 0.1 mg/kg IV/IO.	
2. Rapid sequence intubation. Miller no. 1 blade, 4.5 ETT. **Atropine**, 0.02 mg/kg. **Midazolam** 0.1 mg/kg or **thiopental** 2 to 5 mg/kg IV. **Succinylcholine** 1 to 2 mg/kg IV or **vecuronium** 0.1 to 0.2 mg/kg IV. Cricoid pressure.	Vomits, necessitating suction. Right mainstem intubation. Tube falls out if not properly handled.
3. Place NG and end-tidal CO_2 monitor.	
4. Call for CXR for ETT position.	
5. Gastric lavage and **activated charcoal** 1 g/kg NG.	If patient is not intubated, vomits and aspirates while putting the charcoal down.
6. ECG.	

Repeat Vital Signs

P 200, BP 70/40, bag ventilations.
ECG: Sinus tachycardia, *QRS 130 msec*, right bundle branch block.

Expected Interventions

1. Monitor rhythm.
2. **Lidocaine** 1 mg/kg IV bolus followed by 25 to 50 μg/kg/min continuous infusion.
3. **Sodium bicarbonate** 1 to 2 mEq/kg slow IV push.
4. Establish alternative IV access.
5. Administer **normal saline** 20 ml/kg.

Additional Potential Complications

1. Wide-complex ventricular tachycardia, necessitating cardioversion, or deterioration into asystole, necessitating chest compressions and resuscitation drugs, including epinephrine.

2. Hypotension refractory to fluid bolus, necessitating vasopressors.
3. Recurrent seizures, necessitating benzodiazepines and phenytoin.

Disposition

ICU for further management and monitoring.

Discussion of Objectives

1. *Evaluate and manage altered mental status.*

   The evaluation and management of a child with altered mental status begin with the ABCs. Potential causes to be addressed include head trauma or other intracranial space-occupying lesions resulting in increased intracranial pressure, central nervous system infection, metabolic derangements, hypoxia or hypercarbia, and ingestion of drugs that depress the sensorium.

   This patient had no history of head trauma or localizing CNS signs that would suggest an intracranial process. Also, there was no history of an antecedent illness or fever.

   After oxygenation and placement of appropriate monitors, evaluation should continue with a rapid glucose determination (to rule out hypoglycemia or hyperglycemia) and the administration of **naloxone** for potential opioid ingestions.

   Flumazenil (for a suspected benzodiazepine overdose) should be given *only* after an ECG is obtained to rule out tricyclic antidepressant (TCA) ingestion. Flumazenil may precipitate seizures if given to patients after TCA ingestion.

   Assessment of the airway and gag reflex *before* gastric decontamination is imperative in patients with toxic ingestions. Patients with altered mental status require a mechanical airway before gastric decontamination.

   An ECG is a simple tool that should not be forgotten, especially when a toxic ingestion is being evaluated or considered.

   See Altered Mental Status (p. 193) in Chapter 4.

2. *Recognize the signs and symptoms of TCA overdose.*

   A constellation of *anticholinergic* signs may be present, including dry, flushed skin, blurred vision, large pupils, dry mouth, tachycardia, diminished bowel sounds, confusion, and sedation. The cardiovascular and neurologic systems are the two major systems affected by TCA overdose. *Cardiovascular* toxicity is manifested as sinus tachycardia; conduction disturbances seen on the ECG consist of widened QRS interval, a tall R wave in lead aVR reflecting a rightward shift of QRS axis, and various degrees of AV block. Ventricular dysrhythmias (most commonly ventricular tachycardia), hypotension, and asystole may also occur.

   Altered mental status ranging from delirium to coma and seizures is the major *neurologic* toxic effect.

3. *Manage the complications of TCA overdose.*

   a. Stabilize airway, breathing, and circulation.

   b. Perform gastric decontamination, including lavage and administration of **activated charcoal**. Ensure that the patient's mental status is adequate for protection of his or her airway. Respiratory arrest can occur abruptly and without warning.

   c. Manage seizures by administration of short-acting benzodiazepines initially and **phenytoin** if seizures are recurrent.

d. Cardiotoxicity. For conduction disturbances, administer **sodium bicarbonate** IV initially as a bolus and then as a continuous infusion, aiming for a serum pH of 7.45 to 7.50. The management of ventricular tachycardia and dysrhythmias includes alkalinization with **sodium bicarbonate**, **lidocaine**, and **phenytoin**. Isotonic fluid resuscitation for the initial treatment of hypotension is indicated, but vasopressors should be considered early on because of the risk of late development of acute respiratory distress syndrome (ARDS).

Note: This scenario also works well for an adolescent with altered mental status or seizure who is intoxicated because of a TCA ingestion.

REFERENCES

Boehnhet MT, Lovejoy FH: Value of the QRS duration versus the serum drug level in predicting seizures and ventricular arrhythmias after an acute overdose of tricyclic antidepressants, *N Engl J Med* 313:474-479, 1985.

Foulke GE, Albertson TE, Walby WF: Tricyclic antidepressant overdose: emergency department findings as predictors of clinical course, *Am J Emerg Med* 4:496-500, 1986.

Frommer DA, Kulig KW, Rumack B: Tricyclic antidepressant overdose: a review, *JAMA* 257:521-526, 1987.

18. Altered Mental Status—Diabetic Ketoacidosis

STEPHEN J. TEACH

OBJECTIVES

1. Recognize and manage altered mental status.
2. Recognize the presenting signs and symptoms of diabetic ketoacidosis (DKA).
3. Manage diabetic ketoacidosis.
4. Manage increased intracranial pressure in DKA.

Brief Presenting History

EMTs have brought a 14-year-old male from school with a chief complaint of somnolence.

Initial Vital Signs

P 140, RR 28, BP 70/50.
If asked: T 37° C (ax), estimated weight 50 kg.

Initial Physical Examination

General appearance: Asleep, pale, cool, clammy adolescent with deep, labored respirations. Opens eyes on command. Makes occasional confused verbalizations.
If asked: No evidence of head trauma.
- **Airway:** Patent.
- **Breathing:** Tachypneic but no retractions, breath sounds clear and symmetric, no prolongation of expiratory phase.
- **Circulation:** Heart tones normal but tachycardic, capillary refill time 3 to 4 seconds.
- Pupils 3 to 4 mm, sluggishly reactive.
- Fruity odor of breath.
- Abdomen nondistended and soft.
- No external evidence of trauma.

Further History Given on Request

Patient found by a classmate at school on the floor of the restroom in a pool of emesis. No pills, glue containers, or bottles noted at the scene.
- Past medical history: Negative according to accompanying school nurse.
- Medications: None, NKDA.

Expected interventions	Complications

1. 100% O_2 by face mask.
2. Monitors (ECG, pulse oximeter).
3. Attempt IV access.
   Normal saline 20 ml/kg IV.
4. Laboratory tests: ABG, rapid glucose, CBC, electrolytes, BUN/Cr, UA, ammonia, LFTs, serum and urine toxicologic screen.
5. If glucose level unknown, empiric medications to be considered:
   $D_{25}W$ 1 g/kg (4 ml/kg) IV.
   Naloxone 0.1 mg/kg IV/IM.
   Flumazenil 0.2 mg IV/IM. (See Altered Mental Status [p. 193] in Chapter 4.)
6. 12-Lead ECG (if glucose level unknown).
	If IV access unsuccessful, place a femoral CVL.

Repeat Vital Signs

P 120, RR 28 labored, BP 80/60, O_2 sat 100%, ECG sinus tachycardia.

Progression

No response to initial IV therapy. Becoming less responsive: eye opening to pain only, inappropriate verbalization, withdraws from painful stimuli. GCS 2 + 3 + 4 = 9.

Laboratory Findings

Rapid glucose >500, ABG: pH 7.0, P_{CO_2} 21, P_{O_2} 190, base excess −14.

Expected interventions	Complications
1. Regular **insulin** IV drip 0.1 unit/kg/hr, consider initial regular insulin 0.1 unit/kg IV bolus. 2. Consider further fluid resuscitation with **normal saline** 10 to 20 ml/kg. 3. Consider **$NaHCO_3$** 1 mEq/kg IV over 1 hour. 4. Prepare for rapid sequence intubation.	Vomits, requiring suction. Breathing becomes agonal.

Progression

No eye opening, no verbalization, flexion only to painful stimuli (GCS = 1 + 1 + 3 = 5). Unequal dilated pupils. Decrease in heart rate to 70, blood pressure rises to 140/100.

Expected interventions	Complications
1. Suction, preoxygenate.	
2. Rapid sequence intubation.	Unable to visualize cords if not properly
No. 3 Miller blade, 7.0 cuffed ETT.	suctioned.
Midazolam 0.1 mg/kg IV.	
Succinylcholine 1 to 2 mg/kg IV or	
vecuronium 0.1 to 0.2 mg/kg IV.	
Consider **lidocaine** 1 mg/kg IV.	
Cricoid pressure.	Vomits if no cricoid pressure applied.
Place NG and end-tidal CO_2 monitor.	
3. Hyperventilate, P_{CO_2} 30-35.	Right mainstem intubation.
Repeat ABG.	
4. Reassess fluid management.	Tube falls out if not secured.
Decrease IV fluids if perfusion is adequate.	

Progression

With intubation and increased ICP management the patient's condition stabilizes and pupil size becomes equal.

Disposition

ICU for continued management of increased ICP, ketoacidosis, and relative dehydration.

Potential Complications

This scenario may be made more difficult for advanced participants by making the diagnosis of DKA less evident. Example: A 4-year-old male has a decreased level of consciousness and an occipital scalp laceration after a fall in the bathroom. The fall is the result of DKA-induced dehydration and dizziness, but the differential diagnosis expands to include head trauma, as well as a medicine chest full of ingestion possibilities.

Discussion of Objectives

1. *Recognize and manage altered mental status.*

The differential diagnosis of a patient with an acutely altered mental status includes trauma, toxic ingestions, CNS infections, metabolic abnormalities, hypoxia, hypercapnia, and neurologic impairments. After stabilization of the airway, breathing, and circulation, a thorough assessment of history and physical examination may reveal clues to the etiology.

Standard initial interventions include administration of **glucose** and **naloxone**. **Thiamine** may be indicated in an older adolescent or young adult. If an ingestion is suspected, a trial of **flumazenil** is indicated after the usual contraindications are ruled out. (See Altered Mental Status [p. 193] in Chapter 4.)

The first laboratory study is typically a rapid glucose determination to detect hyperglycemia or hypoglycemia. An ABG is essential for an accurate assessment of acidosis and alkalosis. A toxic screen, including aspirin and acetaminophen levels, and electrolytes with glucose, BUN, and creatinine should be ordered. Ammonia is helpful when the diagnosis of Reye's syndrome is considered. An ECG is used to assess the QRS interval, which may widen in TCA ingestions. A pregnancy test should be obtained for any adolescent female.

2. *Recognize the presenting signs and symptoms of diabetic ketoacidosis.*

The patient in this scenario presents with progressed signs and symptoms of ketoacidosis including Kussmaul breathing, ketotic breath, and altered mental status. In more subtle cases a history of polyuria, polydipsia, and weight loss despite hyperphagia over a period of days to weeks may be presented. Symptoms frequently are precipitated by an intercurrent illness, typically a mild infection, which may confuse the picture. In a patient who has abdominal pain with distention and guarding, hyperpnea, and enuresis, the diagnosis may be confused with an acute abdomen, pneumonia, or a behavioral disorder.

3. *Manage diabetic ketoacidosis.*

The goals of therapy in DKA include the following:

a. Correct dehydration.

b. Reverse acidosis and ketosis.

c. Restore normoglycemia and correct electrolyte abnormalities.

d. Avoid complications of therapy.

Patients in DKA typically are at least 10% dehydrated and may be profoundly dehydrated. Isotonic fluids are indicated in all cases, and more aggressive fluid resuscitation may be necessary to reverse hypotension. An initial 20 ml/kg **normal saline** bolus over the first hour is typically recommended, with slow replacement of the remaining fluid deficit over the next 24 hours. Overzealous replacement of fluid deficit should be avoided.

Replacing vascular volume is essential to improve tissue perfusion and acidosis.

IV **insulin** infusion may begin with an initial bolus of regular insulin 0.1 unit/kg. (*Note:* Bolus insulin therapy is being discontinued at many institutions, especially in younger patients.) A continuous infusion of regular **insulin** 0.08 to 0.1 unit/kg/hr is usually required along with frequent (at least hourly) glucose levels.

In patients with DKA, total body **potassium** is depleted. Therefore potassium should be added to IV fluids after the initial NS bolus.

The use of **sodium bicarbonate** to treat acidosis in DKA remains controversial and is usually reserved for patients with an initial arterial pH less than 7.20.

Overaggressive or improper (hypotonic) fluid resuscitation may precipitate an increase in intracranial pressure caused by cerebral edema. Patients must be closely monitored for headache, change in level of consciousness, vomiting, bradycardia, and hypertension.

4. *Manage increased intracranial pressure in DKA.*

Increased ICP is a devastating complication of DKA. The cause is poorly understood. Most likely it results both from the underlying pathophysiology of DKA and from IV fluid resuscitation management.

The incidence of increased ICP in DKA is less than 1%. It is more common in younger diabetic patients and as an initial presentation of new diabetes.

The best treatment for increased ICP in DKA is prevention. Patients with DKA must be watched closely for changes in level of consciousness or responsiveness that may signal the onset of increased ICP. The fluid management of these patients must be meticulously monitored. See sections on increased intracranial pressure in Chapters 2 and 4 (p. 196).

Note: **Cushing's triad**—bradycardia, hypertension, and abnormal breathing—is a *late* finding of increased ICP and is indicative of impending herniation.

REFERENCES

Hale DE: Endocrine emergencies. In Fleisher GR, Ludwig S, eds: *Textbook of pediatric emergency medicine*, ed 3, Baltimore, 1993, Williams & Wilkins, pp 940-944.

Harris GD et al: Minimizing the risk of brain herniation during treatment of diabetic ketoacidemia: a retrospective study, *J Pediatr* 117:22-31, 1990.

Klekamp J, Churchwell KB: Diabetic ketoacidosis in children: initial clinical assessment and treatment, *Pediatr Ann* 26:387-393, 1996.

Rosenbloom AL: Intracerebral crises during treatment of diabetic ketoacidosis, *Diabetes Care* 13:22-33, 1990.

Saladino RA: Endocrine and metabolic disorders. In Barkin RM: *Pediatric emergency medicine, concepts and clinical practice*, ed 2, St Louis, 1997, Mosby.

Sperling MA: Diabetic ketoacidosis in children. In Lebovitz HE, ed: *Therapy for diabetes mellitus and related disorders*, Falls Church, Va, 1991, American Diabetes Association, pp 36-43.

19. Seizure—Hyponatremia

RICHARD BACHUR

OBJECTIVES

1. Recognize that management of seizures begins with the ABCs.
2. Formulate the differential diagnosis of seizures.
3. Manage seizures caused by hyponatremia.

Brief Presenting History

Option 1: A 2-week-old infant, previously well, has a new onset of seizures. In status epilepticus for approximately 30 minutes.

Option 2: An 8-year-old child, previously well, has a new onset of seizures. In status epilepticus for approximately 30 minutes.

Initial Vital Signs

Option 1: P 180, BP 100/60, RR 86.
If asked: T 37.8°C, estimated weight 4 kg.
Option 2: P 140, BP 140/80, RR irregular and difficult to count.
If asked: T 37.8° C, estimated weight 25 kg.

Initial Physical Examination

Option 1: Large infant lying on a stretcher with tonic-clonic activity of all extremities and grunting respirations.

If asked: Blue-purple discoloration of body.

- **Airway:** Patent, mouth clenched shut, copious secretions.
- **Breathing:** Coarse breath sounds bilaterally.
- **Circulation:** Capillary refill time 3 seconds.
- Anterior fontanel slightly sunken, eyes deviated upward with fine nystagmus, unable to see fundi clearly, no signs of trauma to head or rest of body.
- Abdomen soft.
- Extremities cool.

Option 2: Obese 8-year-old lying supine on stretcher with grunting respirations and tonic-clonic activity of all extremities.

If asked: Blue-purple discoloration of the face.

- **Airway:** Patent, mouth clenched shut, copious secretions.
- **Breathing:** Coarse breath sounds bilaterally.
- **Circulation:** Capillary refill time 3 seconds.
- Neurologic examination: Eyes deviated to right, pupils 5 mm symmetric, minimally reactive, symmetric tonic-clonic activity, teeth clenched.

- No signs of head trauma.
- Abdomen soft.
- Extremities cool.

Further History If Requested

Option 1: Infant was full term, home on second day of life, doing well until 4 days ago when vomiting began. The vomiting has improved since the mother began *diluting the formula.* The infant has had four wet diapers in the last 24 hours. Today the baby has been less vigorous with eating. The baby stiffened during the last feeding. The mother called the EMTs.

Specific points *if asked* individually:
- No trauma.
- No fever.
- Formula was diluted 1:1 with water.
- No family history of neonatal deaths, seizures, or neurologic disease.
- No medicines were given to the baby (and mother is not nursing).

Option 2: Brought in by EMTs from home. Limited history available until parents arrive.
- Previously well, no fever, cough, vomiting, or diarrhea.
- No allergies.
- No prior seizure history.
- No history of ingestion.
- No history of trauma.

Expected interventions	Complications
1. 100% Oxygen by face mask (proper fit). 2. Monitors (ECG and oximeter). 3. IV access attempts. 4. Laboratory tests: Rapid glucose, CBC, electrolytes, calcium, magnesium, phosphorus, blood culture.	Unable to start IV. IO placement necessary.

Progression

With oxygen, the patient's color immediately improves but seizures persist. Capillary refill time is 4 seconds.

Expected interventions	Complications
1. **Diazepam** 0.5 mg/kg PR.	Seizures persist.
2. When IV/IO access obtained: **Lorazepam** 0.1 mg/kg IV/IO or **diazepam** 0.3 mg/kg IV/IO. **Normal saline** 20 ml/kg IV/IO.	
3. Consider load with **phenytoin** 10 mg/kg IV or **phenobarbital** 10 to 20 mg/kg IV.	Cardiovascular collapse if phenytoin given as IV push.
4. Empiric **pyridoxine** 100 mg IV for neonatal seizures.	

Progression

Seizure activity stops, but benzodiazepine therapy results in respiratory suppression and desaturation.

Vital Signs

Option 1: P 200, BP 80/40, RR 8.
Option 2: P 170, BP 140/80, RR 6.

Expected interventions	Complications
1. BVM ventilation with 100% O_2. Cricoid pressure.	No respiratory effort. Vomits if no cricoid pressure applied. Copious secretions, suction required.
2. Rapid sequence intubation. *Option 1:* Miller blade no. 0, ETT 3.5. *Option 2:* Miller blade no. 2, ETT 5.5 cuffed. **Atropine** 0.02 mg/kg IV/IO. Minimum dose 0.1 mg. Cricoid pressure. Place NG and end-tidal CO_2 monitor. CXR for ETT position.	Laryngoscope light out. Right mainstem intubation. If less than minimum dose of atropine given, bradycardia develops. Vomits if no cricoid pressure applied. Tube falls out if not properly handled.
3. ABG.	
4. Consider empiric antibiotics.	

Progression

Parents of *Option 2* arrive: He was previously well except for a "water problem," for which he has been treated with intranasal **DDAVP** (vasopressin) once a day.

Laboratory Findings

Option 1: Rapid glucose 120, Na 120.
Option 2: Rapid glucose 120, Na 112.

Progression

Seizure activity abruptly resumes with generalized tonic-clonic movements.

Expected Interventions

1. **Normal saline** bolus 20 ml/kg IV or **hypertonic saline (3% NaCl** 4 to 6 ml/kg, slow IVP). *Stop* giving hypertonic NaCl with cessation of seizure.

Potential Complications

1. Patient bites tongue, causing bleeding in oropharynx that necessitates use of oral airway or bite block.
2. Instead of respiratory depression leading to intubation, seizure activity persists despite anticonvulsants; tonicity is increased and cyanosis develops, leading to intubation with rapid sequence induction (see p. 10 in Chapter 2).
3. If intubation is delayed for any reason, the patient becomes more cyanotic and the heart rate drops precipitously, resulting ultimately in full arrest.
4. If a phenytoin load is given, it must be infused in normal saline at a rate 1 mg/kg/min. Otherwise dysrhythmias and hypotension will result.
5. The patient is so rigid from the seizure that attempts at positive-pressure ventilation cause pneumothorax.

Disposition

ICU.

Discussion of Objectives

1. *Recognize that management of seizures begins with the ABCs.*
   Maintain the patient's airway, breathing, and circulation. Protect the patient from self-injury during convulsions.
   During a seizure, airway management is complicated by jaw rigidity and secretions. After anticonvulsants have been given, or during the postictal state, airway management can remain complicated because of secretions, occlusion of the airway with the tongue, or depressed gag reflexes. An oral or nasopharyngeal airway may help to support the airway, and suction may be required to prevent aspiration of mucus and saliva.
   Oxygen is administered to prevent hypoxic injury. BVM-assisted respirations may be needed, and in extreme instances or if anticonvulsants cause respiratory suppression, endotracheal intubation may be required.
   Intubation should be performed for the following indications:
   a. Persistent hypoxia despite positive-pressure ventilation by BVM.
   b. Hemodynamic compromise.
   c. Increased intracranial pressure (i.e., suspected closed head injuries or meningitis).
   Paralytics must be used in a cyanotic patient who cannot open his or her mouth or ventilate because of chest wall rigidity. In addition, paralytic agents with proper sedation (and lidocaine) are essential if increased intracranial pressure is a concern. Neurologic findings should be noted

before paralytics are given. If the patient is intubated because of respiratory compromise from anticonvulsant therapy, paralytics are not typically used.

Coincident with assessment of the airway and breathing, cardiac monitoring, oximetry, and attempts at IV access are begun. Regarding "circulation," the sequence of hypertension and tachycardia followed by hypotension and bradycardia when seizures are prolonged is expected. Hypotension may also result from an underlying process such as dehydration or associated hypoglycemia or hyponatremia. Access is important to support the circulation with isotonic crystalloid fluid replacement and to deliver anticonvulsants, glucose, or sodium. Occasionally, as in patients with septic shock, inotropic support may be required.

The secondary survey should be performed once the ABCs have been addressed to identify other possible etiologies of seizure activity.

Hyperthermia may result from prolonged seizure activity and must be treated aggressively with antipyretics and external cooling measures such as cooling blankets.

During a seizure it is important to shield the child from injury induced by the violence of the convulsions. Position the patient on his or her side (to maintain a patent airway) on a soft surface to protect the head from banging.

See Seizures (p. 195) in Chapter 4 and mock code 21, Seizure—Status Epilepticus (p. 107).

2. *Formulate the differential diagnosis of seizures.*

The challenge in treating seizures is to simultaneously stabilize the patient, direct therapy, and conduct a diagnostic evaluation to uncover the etiology of the seizure (Table 3-2).

Table 3-2   *Diagnostic Evaluation for Etiology of Seizures*

Etiology	Laboratory or radiologic study
CNS infection	CBC, blood culture, and CSF analysis
Trauma, suspected abuse	CT of head, cervical spine films
Metabolic: hyponatremia, hypoglycemia, vomiting, diarrhea, dehydration, inborn errors of metabolism	Rapid glucose determination, electrolytes with calcium and phosphorus, BUN/Cr, UA, ammonia, metabolic screen
Ingestions	Anion gap, toxicologic screen, ECG
Anoxia, hypoxia	Pulse oximeter, ABG
Known seizure disorders	Anticonvulsant levels
Intracranial lesion: tumor, abscess, CVA, AVM	CT or MRI of the head

Hypoglycemia can be manifested as a spectrum of symptoms from lethargy to seizure or coma. Potential causes of hypoglycemia include:

a. Sepsis, most commonly in infants.

b. Decreased intake caused by acute illness, especially in infants.

c. Poor absorption related to vomiting and diarrhea.

d. Inborn errors of metabolism.

   e. Poisonings such as those by alcohols, salicylates, propranolol, insulin overdose, and ingestion of oral hypoglycemic agents.

   f. Fulminant liver failure, Reye's syndrome.

3. *Manage seizures secondary to hyponatremia.*

Precipitous drops in serum sodium concentration lead to neurologic dysfunction, including seizures. Typical causes are syndrome of inappropriate antidiuretic hormone secretion (SIADH), water intoxication, and renal failure. Seizures caused by hyponatremia often remain refractory to therapy until the serum sodium level is elevated. Rapid correction can be achieved with hypertonic saline. Giving hypertonic saline, **3% NaCl** 4 to 6 ml/kg as slow IV push, typically raises serum sodium levels by 5 mEq/L. The goal is cessation of the seizure.

Once the seizure has stopped, serum sodium concentrations can be corrected slowly (usually through fluid restriction with free water diuresis). Excessive, immediate correction should be avoided because of the potential complication of central pontine and extrapontine myelinolysis. In the absence of seizures, serum sodium may be corrected by infusion of **normal saline**.

REFERENCES

Avner ED: Clinical disorders of water metabolism: hyponatremia and hypernatremia, *Pediatr Ann* 24:23-30, 1995.

Ayus JC, Krothapalli RK, Arieff AI: Treatment of symptomatic hyponatremia and its relationship to brain damage, *N Engl J Med* 317:1190-1195, 1987.

Sarnaik AP et al: Management of hyponatremic seizures in children with hypertonic saline: a safe and effective strategy, *Crit Care Med* 19:758-762, 1991.

20. Seizure—Hypoglycemia

FRANCES W. CRAIG

OBJECTIVES

1. Recognize that management of seizures begins with the ABCs.
2. Formulate the differential diagnosis of seizures.
3. Manage seizures secondary to hypoglycemia.

Brief Presenting History

An 18-month-old male brought in by his parents is unresponsive and is moving his arms and legs rhythmically.

Initial Vital Signs

HR 180, RR 36, BP 65/40.
If asked: T 36.0° C (R), estimated weight 12 kg.

Initial Physical Examination

General appearance: Generalized tonic-clonic movements of upper and lower extremities.
If asked: Shallow, fast breathing with occasional episodes of transient apnea. Breath sounds clear bilaterally.

- **Airway:** Patent, teeth clenched, copious secretions.
- **Breathing:** Breath sounds full, coarse bilaterally.
- **Circulation:** Heart rate and rhythm regular, pulses weak bilaterally. Perioral cyanosis, capillary refill time 4 seconds.
- Head atraumatic. Pupils 3 mm bilaterally, sluggishly reactive to light.
- Extremities without evidence of trauma.

Further History Given on Request

- The child has been in his grandfather's care over the weekend.
- No history of fever, vomiting, or diarrhea.
- Past medical history negative, no medications.
- The grandfather is taking daily oral medications for non-insulin-dependent diabetes.

Expected interventions	Complications
1. 100% oxygen, head in midline. BVM-assisted ventilation. Suction as needed.	Vomits.
2. IV access.	IV attempts unsuccessful, necessitating IO placement.
Normal saline 20 ml/kg IV/IO.	
3. Laboratory tests: Rapid glucose, ABG, electrolytes, CBC, blood culture.	
4. **Lorazepam** 0.05 to 0.1 mg/kg IV/IO.	Persistent seizure.
5. Repeat **lorazepam** 0.05 to 0.1 mg/kg IV/IO.	

Repeat Vital Signs

HR 140, RR 4, BP 70/P.

Laboratory Findings

Rapid glucose 25.

Expected interventions	Complications
1. BVM-assisted ventilation with 100% oxygen. Cricoid pressure.	Vomits if no cricoid pressure used.
2. Prepare for rapid sequence intubation.	
3. $D_{25}W$ 2 to 4 ml/kg IV/IO.	PIV infiltrates if $D_{50}W$ given.

Progression

Seizure activity stops, patient now apneic. Capillary refill time 4 seconds.

Expected interventions	Complications
1. Rapid sequence intubation. 4.5 or 5.0 ETT, Miller no. 1 blade. **Atropine** 0.02 mg/kg IV/IO. Cricoid pressure. Place NG and end-tidal CO_2 monitor. CXR for ETT position.	Right mainstem intubation. Desaturation, pulse oximeter 88%. Vomits if no cricoid pressure applied. Extubated if ETT not handled properly.
2. Repeat **normal saline** 20 ml/kg IV/IO.	IO infiltrates.
3. Attempt femoral CVL.	
4. Repeat rapid glucose.	
5. Foley catheter.	
6. **Activated charcoal** 1 g/kg NG.	

Progression

GTC seizure activity begins again, rapid glucose 20.

Expected interventions	Complications
1. **Lorazepam** 0.05 to 0.1 mg/kg IV/IO.	Patient is extubated if not rapidly sedated or paralyzed.
2. **D$_{25}$W** 2 to 4 ml/kg IV/IO. Begin continuous **dextrose** infusion. 3. Consider **pancuronium** 0.1 mg/kg IV.	

Potential Complications

1. Intubation is unsuccessful and asystole develops, necessitating BVM ventilation and chest compressions.
2. Oral hypoglycemic ingestion goes unrecognized, and seizure activity persists.

Disposition

ICU for management of seizures and hypoglycemia.

Discussion of Objectives

1. *Recognize that management of seizures begins with the ABCs.*
   Maintain the patient's airway, breathing, and circulation. Protect the patient from self-injury during convulsions.
   During a seizure, airway management is complicated by jaw rigidity and secretions. After anticonvulsants have been given, or during the postictal state, airway management can remain complicated because of secretions, occlusion of the airway with the tongue, or depressed gag reflexes. An oral or nasopharyngeal airway may help to maintain a patent airway, and suction may be required to prevent aspiration of mucus and saliva.
   Oxygen is administered to prevent hypoxic injury. BVM-assisted respirations may be needed, and in extreme instances or if respiratory suppression occurs secondary to administration of anticonvulsants, endotracheal intubation may be required.
   Intubation should be performed for the following indications:
   a. Persistent hypoxia despite positive-pressure ventilation by BVM.
   b. Hemodynamic compromise.
   c. Increased intracranial pressure (e.g., because of suspected closed head injuries or meningitis).
   Paralytic agents must be used in cyanotic patients if practitioners are unable to open the the patient's mouth or ventilate because of chest wall rigidity. In addition, paralytics with proper sedation (and lidocaine) are essential if increased intracranial pressure is a concern. The neurologic findings should be noted before paralytics are given. If the patient is intubated because of respiratory compromise from anticonvulsant therapy, paralytics are not typically used.
   Coincident with assessment of the airway and breathing, cardiac monitoring, oximetry, and

attempts at IV access are begun. Regarding "circulation," the sequence of hypertension and tachycardia followed by hypotension and bradycardia when seizures are prolonged is expected. Hypotension may also result from an underlying process such as dehydration or associated hypoglycemia or hyponatremia. Access is important to support the circulation with isotonic fluid replacement and to deliver anticonvulsants, glucose, or sodium. Occasionally, as in patients with septic shock, inotropic support may be required.

The secondary survey should be performed once access has been achieved to identify other possible causes of seizure activity.

Hyperthermia may result from prolonged seizure activity and must be addressed aggressively with antipyretics and external cooling measures such as cooling blankets.

During a seizure it is important to protect the child from injury induced by the violence of the convulsions. Position the patient on his or her side (to maintain a patent airway) on a soft surface to protect the head from banging.

See Seizures (p. 195) in Chapter 4 and mock code 21, Seizure—Status Epilepticus (p. 107).

2. *Formulate the differential diagnosis of seizures.*

The challenge of treating seizures is to simultaneously stabilize the patient, direct therapy, and conduct a diagnostic evaluation that will uncover the etiology of the seizure (Table 3-3).

Table 3-3   *Diagnostic Evaluation for Etiology of Seizures*

Etiology	Laboratory or radiologic study
CNS infection	CBC, blood culture, and CSF analysis
Trauma, suspected abuse	CT of head, cervical spine films
Metabolic: hyponatremia, hypoglycemia, vomiting, diarrhea, dehydration, inborn errors of metabolism	Rapid glucose determination, electrolytes with calcium and phosphorus, BUN/Cr, UA, ammonia, metabolic screen
Ingestions	Anion gap, toxicologic screen, ECG
Anoxia, hypoxia	Pulse oximeter, ABG
Known seizure disorders	Anticonvulsant levels
Intracranial lesion: tumor, abscess, CVA, AVM	CT or MRI of the head

Hypoglycemia presents with a spectrum of symptoms from lethargy to seizure or coma. Infants with immature livers and decreased ability to make glucose from stores of glycogen are especially susceptible to hypoglycemia when stressed.

Potential causes of hypoglycemia include:

a. Sepsis, most commonly in infants.

b. Decreased intake because of acute illness, especially in infants or children with chronic disease.

c. Poor absorption owing to vomiting and diarrhea.

d. Inborn errors of metabolism.

e. Poisonings such as those caused by alcohols, salicylates, propranolol, insulin overdose, and ingestion of oral hypoglycemic agents.

f. Fulminant liver failure, Reye's syndrome.

3. *Manage seizures caused by hypoglycemia.*

Seizures caused by hypoglycemia must be treated with rapid infusion of dextrose. A 25% dextrose solution as D_{25} water may be pushed through a peripheral IV. The dose is 0.5 to 1 g/kg, which is 2 to 4 ml/kg of $D_{25}W$. Greater concentrations such as 50% dextrose ($D_{50}W$) may not be given through a PIV because the high solute concentration leads to tissue infiltration. Infants may be given $D_{10}W$ 5 to 10 ml/kg IV. After initial treatment it is important to recheck glucose levels frequently. Persistent hypoglycemia may require a continuous dextrose infusion.

REFERENCES

Aynsley-Green A: Hypoglycemia in infants and children, *Clin Endocr Metab* 11:159-193, 1982.

Haymond MW: Hypoglycemia in infants and children, *Endocrinol Metab Clin North Am* 18:211-252, 1989.

Segeleon JE, Haun S: Status epilepticus in children, *Pediatric Ann* 25:380-386, 1996.

21. Seizure—Status Epilepticus

JOE WATHEN

OBJECTIVES
1. Recognize the patient in status epilepticus.
2. Differentiate the possible etiologies of status epilepticus.
3. Identify the key management issues in treating status epilepticus.

Brief Presenting History

A 4-year-old boy with cerebral palsy, developmental delay, and a seizure disorder is brought in with a generalized tonic-clonic seizure. He had 10 minutes of seizure activity before the paramedics arrived. He received 2 mg rectal **diazepam** en route after IV attempts in the field were unsuccessful. He arrives with blow-by oxygen and continued seizure activity. Seizure activity has now lasted a total of 30 to 40 minutes.

Initial Vital Signs

HR 160, RR 28, BP 88/50.
If asked: T 38.5° C (R), estimated weight 12 kg (smaller than expected for age because of chronic disease).

Initial Physical Examination

General appearance: Generalized tonic-clonic seizure activity, eyes rolled back, gurgling breath sounds, pale skin color, copious oral secretions.
If asked: No focal neurologic findings, no signs of trauma.
• **Airway:** Patent.
• **Breathing:** Coarse breath sounds bilaterally.
• **Circulation:** Capillary refill time 3 seconds.
• Seizure involves all extremities, eyes deviated to the left.

Further History Given on Request

The patient's epilepsy was diagnosed at 6 months of age. He has been receiving **carbamazepine** and **valproic acid** since that time. He usually has a seizure lasting 3 to 5 minutes every few months. His last seizure was 2 weeks ago. He has missed his last two doctor's appointments, and no recent anticonvulsant levels are known.
• He has had upper respiratory symptoms and low-grade fever for the last 3 days.
• NKDA, taking no other medications, no known ingestions.
• There is no history of trauma. Before the seizure he had been acting normally.

Expected interventions	Complications
1. Assess ABCs.	Airway compromise.
2. 100% oxygen, suction the oropharynx.	
3. Cardiac monitor, pulse oximeter.	
4. Establish IV access. **Normal saline** 20 ml/kg IV or IO.	IV access unsuccessful, necessitating PR medications or IO placement.
5. Laboratory tests: Rapid glucose, electrolytes, anticonvulsant levels.	
6. **Lorazepam** 0.05 to 0.1 mg/kg IV or IO or **diazepam** 0.5 mg/kg PR.	

Repeat Vital Signs

HR 175, RR 20, BP 80/45.

Laboratory Findings

Rapid glucose 178.

Progression

Patient continues to have GTC seizure; now 50 minutes in length.

Expected interventions	Complications
1. Establish IV or IO access.	
2. **Lorazepam** 0.1 mg/kg IV or IO.	Persistent seizure activity.
3. Load with **phenytoin** 15 to 20 mg/kg IV or IO (not to exceed 1 mg/kg/min) or **phenobarbital** 10 to 20 mg/kg IV or IO.	Rapid phenytoin load leads to cardiovascular collapse.* If phenobarbital used, patient becomes apneic.
4. Contact neurology service.	
Note: Benzodiazepines can be repeated every 5 minutes for total of four doses.	

*__Fosphenytoin__ can now be given over 5 minutes without hemodynamic compromise.

Laboratory Results

Carbamazepine level 2 mg/dl (therapeutic level 4 to 12 mg/dl), valproic acid level 30 mg/dl (50 to 100 mg/dl). Na 138, K 4.3, HCO_3 18, BUN 7, Cr 0.4.

Progression	Expected interventions	Complications
Option 1 Seizure stops, patient becomes apneic. Poor air movement with BVM.	1. Rapid sequence intubation. **Atropine** 0.02 mg/kg IV. **Succinylcholine** 1 mg/kg IV. Miller no. 2 blade, 5.0 ETT. Cricoid pressure. Place NG and end-tidal CO_2. CXR for ETT position.	Vomits if no cricoid pressure or NG tube.
Option 2 Patient continues to have seizure activity.	1. Load additional **phenytoin** 10 mg/kg IV. Add **phenobarbital** 20 mg/kg IV. 2. Rapid sequence intubation. **Atropine** 0.02 mg/kg IV. **Succinylcholine** 1 mg/kg IV. Miller no. 2 blade, 5.0 ETT. Cricoid pressure. Place NG and end-tidal CO_2. CXR for ETT position. 3. Additional anticonvulsant therapy. **Midazolam** or **lidocaine** continuous IV infusion, or **pentobarbital**-induced coma.	Persistent seizure. Vomits if no cricoid pressure or NG tube.
Option 3 Seizure stops, capillary refill time 4 seconds, T 41.4° C.	1. Repeat **normal saline** 20 ml/kg IV. 2. **Acetaminophen** 15 mg/kg PR, cooling blankets. 3. Consider inotropes. **Dopamine** 5 to 10 μg/kg/min.	Persistent hypotension despite additional fluids.

◆

Additional Potential Complications

1. Hyperthermia and hypotension lead to cardiovascular collapse.
2. Continued seizure activity without proper sedation leads to extubation.
3. Failure to administer oxygen properly and control the airway leads to anoxia and asystole.

Disposition

ICU, neurology consult, possible general anesthesia (**halothane, pentobarbital** coma) and EEG monitoring.

Discussion of Objectives

(See Seizures [p. 195] in Chapter 4.)

1. *Recognize the patient in status epilepticus (SE).*

   Status epilepticus is defined as continuous seizure activity for at least 30 minutes or repeated seizures in which the patient does not return to baseline mental status. SE is classified as either generalized or partial. Generalized SE is considered as either convulsive or nonconvulsive (absence/atonic). Partial SE is divided into simple (normal consciousness) and complex (clouded consciousness or unconsciousness).

   Each year in the United States SE occurs in 60,000 to 120,000 persons, with the majority of episodes occurring in children. Among children who develop epilepsy before the first year of life, 70% will have an episode of SE. Among all persons with epilepsy, 20% have an episode of SE within a 5-year period. Morbidity can be significant with SE and may include anoxia, hyperthermia, aspiration, metabolic acidosis, rhabdomyolysis, renal failure, and neurologic damage. Mortality ranges from 4% to 30% with recent decreases secondary to improved supportive care and pharmacotherapy.

2. *Differentiate the possible etiologies of status epilepticus.*

   The challenge in treating SE is to simultaneously stabilize the patient, direct therapy, and conduct a diagnostic evaluation to uncover the etiology (Table 3-4).

Table 3-4 *Diagnostic Evaluation for Etiology of Status Epilepticus*

Etiology	Laboratory or radiologic study
CNS infection	CBC, blood culture, and CSF analysis
Trauma, suspected abuse	CT of head, cervical spine films
Metabolic: hypoglycemia, hyponatremia	Rapid glucose determination, electrolytes with calcium and phosphorus, BUN/Cr, UA
Vomiting, diarrhea, dehydration, inborn error of metabolism	Ammonia, metabolic screen
Ingestions	Anion gap, toxicologic screen, ECG
Anoxia/hypoxia	Pulse oximeter, ABG
Known seizure disorders	Anticonvulsant levels
Intracranial lesion: tumor, abscess, CVA, AVM	CT or MRI of the head

One fourth of childhood SE is idiopathic, one fourth is idiopathic with fever, and one fourth is related to a congenital or developmental neurologic abnormality or a previous CNS insult (e.g., traumatic brain injury, stroke, or meningitis). In the remaining one fourth of children with SE the cause is an acute event such as trauma, anoxia, metabolic abnormality, toxin exposure, intracranial hemorrhage, tumor, CNS infection, or anticonvulsant medication withdrawal.

Neonatal seizures are usually due to perinatal hypoxic encephalopathy, structural brain abnormalities, inborn errors of metabolism, electrolyte abnormalities, or pyridoxine deficiency.

In older children the causes of SE include febrile seizure, trauma, and accidental overdoses. In adolescents SE is usually idiopathic or similar to adult patterns (i.e., related to trauma, anticonvulsant medication withdrawal, or alcohol or drug abuse).

3. *Identify the key management issues in treating status epilepticus.*

Management of status epilepticus is based on three principles:

a. Maintain the patient's ABCs.

An oral or nasopharyngeal airway may be helpful to support the airway, and suction may be necessary to prevent aspiration of mucus and saliva. BVM-assisted respirations may be needed, and in extreme instances or if respiratory suppression results from administration of anticonvulsants, endotracheal intubation may be required.

Hypotension may be caused by an underlying process such as dehydration or may develop after prolonged seizure activity and requires isotonic fluid replacement. Occasionally, as in patients with septic shock, inotropic support may be required.

Hyperthermia may result from prolonged SE and must be addressed aggressively with antipyretics and external cooling measures such as cooling blankets.

During SE it is important to protect the child from injury caused by the violence of convulsions. Position the patient on his or her side (to prevent aspiration) on a soft surface to protect the head from banging.

b. Be familiar with the pharmacologic options to stop and prevent further convulsions. Benzodiazepines remain the initial drug of choice. **Lorazepam** 0.05 to 0.1 mg/kg provides a longer duration of action then **diazepam** or **midazolam**. **Diazepam** may be given rectally, 0.2 to 0.5 mg/kg. Phenytoin is the preferred second drug of choice because of the reduced respiratory depression and sedation as compared with **phenobarbital**. The recent approval of **fosphenytoin** allows for a significantly more rapid administration without the serious cardiovascular side effects. **Fosphenytoin** dosage is expressed in phenytoin equivalents (PE). The loading dose for emergency use is 15 to 20 mg/kg (PE) IV. There is an increased risk of respiratory depression, which may necessitate endotracheal intubation and mechanical ventilation, when both benzodiazepines and phenobarbital are used.

If an infant is having a seizure without an apparent etiology, **pyridoxine** 100 mg IV should be given empirically for presumed vitamin B_6 deficiency.

Inadequate dosage of anticonvulsant drugs remains one of the most frequent errors in providing initial therapy for SE. When treating SE the practitioner should always be prepared to control the airway because most acute anticonvulsant therapies suppress respiration. When the patient is being intubated, short-term paralytics should be used to avoid masking ongoing seizure activity.

c. Establish the etiology of SE with specific treatment as indicated. Seizure activity may require treatment with glucose, sodium, calcium, or pyridoxine for underlying deficiencies. Many ingestions have specific antidotes. Traumatic injuries and space-occupying lesions may require emergency surgery.

REFERENCES

Appleton R et al: Lorazepam versus diazepam in the acute treatment of epileptic seizures and status epilepticus, *Dev Med Child Neurol* 37:682-688, 1995.

Pellock JM: Status epilepticus in children: update and review, *J Child Neurol* 9:27-35, 1994.

Roberts MR, Eng-Bourquin J: Status epilepticus in children, *Emerg Med Clin North Am* 13:489-507, 1995.

Segeleon JE, Haun S: Status epilepticus in children, *Pediatric Ann* 25:380-386, 1996.

Stores G et al: Non-convulsive status epilepticus, *Arch Dis Child* 73:106-111, 1995.

22. Headache—Hypertensive Emergency

KATHRYN D. CLARK

OBJECTIVES
1. Recognize hypertension in a pediatric patient.
2. Recognize and treat a hypertensive emergency.
3. Manage hypertensive encephalopathy.

Brief Presenting History

A 9-year-old child is brought for treatment with the chief complaint of headache of 4 days' duration. The headache is worse this morning, and the patient now complains of dizziness and blurry vision.

Initial Vital Signs

P 130, BP 140/110, RR 22.
If asked: T 37.8° C (T), estimated weight 30 kg.

Initial Physical Examination

General appearance: Pale, quiet, holding head in hands.
If asked: Oriented to person, not to place, unable to follow commands.
- **Airway:** Patent, speaks clearly.
- **Breathing:** Lungs clear, no crackles or rales.
- **Circulation:** Slight tachycardia, no murmurs, capillary refill time 2 seconds, symmetric, strong distal pulses, no bruits, four extremity blood pressures are approximately equal 140s/110s.
- HEENT: Periorbital edema, pupils equal and reactive, discs sharp, arteriolar constriction, no retinal hemorrhages.
- Pharynx clear, no erythema or exudate.
- Abdomen nondistended, no palpable masses, no hepatosplenomegaly, no costovertebral angle tenderness.
- Neurologic examination nonfocal, vision too blurry for visual acuity.
- No external signs of trauma.

Further History Given on Request

The patient had a sore throat 2 weeks earlier that resolved spontaneously after 2 to 3 days. The patient has had slightly decreased oral intake. Parents are unaware of any change in urinary pattern. No previous history of headaches.
- No history of trauma or ingestion.
- The patient is not on routine medications and has NKDA.

Expected interventions	Complications
1. Oxygen, quiet, comfort, elevate head of bed. 2. Monitors (ECG, pulse oximeter). 3. Check sphygmomanometer cuff size. 4. IV access—no fluids. 5. Laboratory tests: electrolytes, BUN/Cr, UA/UC, CBC, strep screen. 6. **Nifedipine** 0.25 to 0.5 mg/kg SL.	If IV fluids given, congestive heart failure or pulmonary edema develops.

Repeat Vital Signs

P 109, BP 130/100, RR 22, pulse oximeter 97%.

Progression

Generalized tonic-clonic seizure activity develops.

Expected interventions	Complications
1. **Diazoxide** 3 to 5 mg/kg IVP. 2. **Lorazepam** 0.05 to 0.1 mg/kg IV.	Seizure persists.

Progression

Seizure activity stops.

Laboratory Results

Sodium 135, potassium 3.7, chloride 93, bicarbonate 25, BUN 53, Cr 2.2, Hct 40.
UA specific gravity 1.009, pH 7.5, 2+ protein, 3+ blood, red cells too numerous to count, 0-2 granular casts, 0-5 red cell casts.
Strep screen positive.

Expected Interventions

1. Contact renal service.
2. **Penicillin** 100,000 units/kg IV.

Additional Potential Complications

1. Apnea develops after patient receives lorazepam.
2. Left ventricular failure occurs from fluid overload if a bolus is given.
3. Hyperkalemia develops as a result of renal failure.
4. Hypotension develops because of overaggressive antihypertensive medications.

Disposition

ICU for continued management and monitoring of hypertension.

Discussion of Objectives

1. *Recognize hypertension in a pediatric patient.*

   Although relatively uncommon in the pediatric population, hypertension is an important cause of morbidity. Hypertension is defined as systolic, diastolic, or mean arterial pressure greater than the 95th percentile for age. Significant hypertension is blood pressure measurements persistently between the 95th and 99th percentiles for age and sex. Severe hypertension is blood pressure at or above the 99th percentile or any blood pressure affecting end organs.

   Using a proper size pediatric blood pressure cuff is important. The bladder should be two thirds of the length of upper arm and must encompass the circumference of the arm.

   Patients with new onset of mild to moderate hypertension may have no symptoms or only mild complaints of headache, vomiting, abdominal pain, epistaxis, or irritability. Malignant hypertension with acute significant changes in blood pressure is manifested much more dramatically. New murmurs, congestive heart failure, lower motor neuron facial palsies, or hematuria may be found.

2. *Recognize and treat a hypertensive emergency.*

   Hypertensive urgency is a state of severely elevated blood pressure that is potentially harmful, although there is no evidence of end-organ damage or dysfunction. Conversely, a hypertensive emergency exists when elevated blood pressure is associated with evidence of secondary organ damage. Secondary or end-organ involvement may be manifest as hypertensive encephalopathy or acute left ventricular failure.

   Management of hypertension begins with support of the ABCs. The blood pressure should be lowered promptly but gradually. The mean arterial pressure is reduced by approximately 25% over minutes to hours, depending on the etiology and extent of involvement. Hypertensive patients with headaches and vomiting may have their blood pressure lowered over hours, whereas patients having seizures or with impending herniation should have alleviation of hypertension over a few minutes.

   In the treatment of acute hypertension, careful monitoring for hypotension and neurologic deficits is important. Drug therapy options to be considered based on route and onset of action are listed below.

   Nifedipine is a calcium channel blocker that is given sublingually or orally and has an onset of action of 30 to 60 minutes. It reduces peripheral vascular resistance without affecting cardiac output.

   Diazoxide is given by rapid IV push and has a rapid onset of action, 1 to 5 minutes. It is a potent hypotensive agent.

   Sodium nitroprusside is given as a continuous IV infusion and has an immediate onset of action. Indwelling arterial monitoring is recommended when this drug is used. It is contraindicated in renal insufficiency.

   Labetalol may also be given as a continuous IV infusion, but its onset of action is slower, about 5 minutes, and it is not as potent a hypotensive agent as nitroprusside.

3. *Manage hypertensive encephalopathy.*

   In hypertensive encephalopathy, autoregulation of cerebral blood flow is disrupted, which leads to either:

   a. Overregulation with exaggerated vasospasm and ischemic injury or

   b. Underregulation with increased cerebral flow and cerebral edema.

   No single symptom or sign is diagnostic. Symptoms include nausea and vomiting, headaches, altered mental status, visual disturbances, seizures, and stroke. The diagnosis is confirmed by rapid improvement after a decrease in blood pressure. The differential diagnosis of hypertensive encephalopathy includes:

   a. Head trauma.

   b. Cerebral hemorrhage or infarction.

   c. Meningitis, encephalitis.

   d. Brain tumor.

   e. Uremic encephalopathy.

   Treatment is aimed at reducing blood pressure rapidly. For this reason diazoxide and nitroprusside are considered first-line therapies. Seizures may be resistant to traditional therapy with benzodiazepines. Seizure control is unlikely until hypertension is controlled.

Additional Comments

1. In the scenario offered above in which hypertension results from acute renal failure caused by poststreptococcal glomerulonephritis, fluid overload may exacerbate hypertension. **Furosemide** to initiate diuresis is another method of treating hypertension in this situation.

2. If sodium nitroprusside is used on a long-term basis, levels of cyanide produced by metabolites must be monitored.

REFERENCES

Calhoun DA, Oparil S: Treatment of hypertensive crisis, *N Engl J Med* 323:1177-1183, 1990.

Deal JE, Barratt TM, Dillon MJ: Management of hypertensive emergencies, *Arch Dis Child* 67:1089-1092, 1992.

Farine M, Arbus GS: Management of hypertensive emergencies in children, *Pediatr Emerg Care* 5:51-55, 1989.

Groshong T: Hypertensive crisis in children, *Pediatr Ann* 25:368-376, 1996.

CARDIAC EMERGENCIES
23. Supraventricular Tachycardia
ANDREW ATZ

OBJECTIVES
1. Distinguish supraventricular tachycardia (SVT) from sinus tachycardia.
2. Manage SVT without hemodynamic compromise.
3. Recognize situations in which aggressive management of SVT is indicated.

Brief Presenting History

A 6-year-old boy has an obvious deformity of the right forearm after falling off his bike. He complains of dizziness and pounding in his chest.

Initial Vital Signs

P 245, BP unable to register, RR 22.
If asked: T 36.9° C oral, estimated weight 25 kg, pulse oximetry 97% in room air.

Initial Physical Examination

General appearance: Anxious, complaining of right arm pain, otherwise very alert.
If asked:
- **Airway:** Patent.
- **Breathing:** Clear breath sounds with no retractions.
- **Circulation:** Tachycardic, normal S_1 and S_2, no murmur, pulse strong, capillary refill time 2 to 3 seconds.
- No evidence of other trauma.
- No hepatosplenomegaly.
- No peripheral edema.

Further History Given on Request

The patient was wearing his helmet, no loss of consciousness.
- Healthy child, no hospitalizations. No prior history of rhythm abnormalities.
- No medications, NKDA.
- Family history negative.

Expected interventions	Complications
1. 100% O_2.	
2. Monitors (ECG, oximeter).	
3. Monitor blood pressure.	Unable to register BP with this heart rate.
4. IV access.	
Normal saline 20 ml/kg bolus IV.	Difficulty starting IV.
5. 12-Lead electrocardiogram.	
6. Splint arm, consider pain medications.	
Morphine 0.1 mg/kg IV.	

Progression

After bolus of fluid 20 ml/kg crystalloid and splinting of the arm the patient remains anxious and dizzy. No change in heart rate. Pulses strong, unable to obtain a blood pressure. The 12-lead ECG reveals very regular narrow-complex tachycardia at 245 beats per minute (see Appendix E, p. 218).

Expected Interventions

First-line therapy, without drugs:
1. Increase vagal tone maneuvers.
2. Cover face with bag of ice to evoke "diving reflex."
3. Direct patient to perform Valsalva maneuver.
4. For infants, try nasal suction or rectal stimulation.
5. Call cardiology department.

Progression	Expected interventions
Option 1 Heart rate converts to sinus rhythm with vagal maneuvers.	1. Obtain a 12-lead ECG while patient is in sinus rhythm. 2. Continue cardiac monitoring. 3. Consult cardiology department.
Option 2 Patient becomes more anxious. All efforts to lower heart rate fail.	1. **Adenosine** 0.05 mg/kg IV; if unsuccessful repeat **adenosine** 0.1, 0.2 mg/kg IV.
Option 3 Patient becomes acutely dyspneic, diaphoretic, and poorly responsive. Capillary refill time is 4 seconds. See Tachycardia (p. 200) in Chapter 4.	1. Synchronized cardioversion, 0.5 to 1 J/kg. If patient is awake, sedate with **midazolam** 0.1 mg/kg IV.

Additional Potential Complications

1. Patient converts to normal sinus rhythm briefly but then returns to SVT, requiring repeat treatment with adenosine.
2. A hemodynamically uncompromised patient has persistent SVT despite adenosine 0.2 mg/kg given twice, requiring involvement of cardiology for external pacing.

Disposition

If patient is responsive to vagal maneuvers or adenosine, consult cardiology. If patient is unresponsive to noninvasive measures, admit for further therapy and observation.

Discussion of Objectives

1. *Distinguish supraventricular tachycardia (SVT) from sinus tachycardia.*
   Supraventricular tachycardia is a reentrant type of tachycardia. In reentrant tachycardia the onset and cessation are abrupt and the rate is highly regular. Unlike sinus tachycardias, SVT is not responsive to analgesia or sedation, volume resuscitation, or control of fever. An ECG reveals a regular, narrow-complex tachycardia, typically greater than 240 beats per minute.
2. *Manage SVT without hemodynamic compromise.*
   Many reentrant tachycardias can be managed with maneuvers to increase vagal tone. For some children who have infrequent episodes the Valsalva maneuver can be used at home. A bag of ice placed on the face will convert the rhythm in some children, especially infants. Use of ocular compression should be discouraged in the pediatric population because of possible retinal injury. **Adenosine** is an effective treatment for SVT in many cases. The dose is 0.05 mg/kg IV, which is doubled to 0.1 mg/kg if not initially effective. A third dose of 0.2 mg/kg may be administered and repeated for resistant SVT. Adenosine is an extremely volatile drug that must be given by rapid intravenous push followed immediately by a saline flush to be effective. If effective, adenosine will block conduction at the AV node and may (only transiently) cause profound but asymptomatic bradycardia.
3. *Recognize situations in which aggressive management of SVT is indicated.*
   At any point if the patient becomes hypotensive or experiences altered mental status because of compromised blood flow to the brain, synchronized cardioversion should be administered. (See Tachycardia [p. 200] in Chapter 4.)

Additional Comments

1. After the SVT rhythm is corrected, a 12-lead ECG should be obtained to differentiate Wolff-Parkinson-White from other reentrant tachycardias.

REFERENCES

Fyler DC, ed: *Nadas' pediatric cardiology*, Philadelphia, 1992, Hanley & Belfus, pp 377-415.

Ralston MA, Knilans TK, Hannon DW, Daniels SR: Use of adenosine for diagnosis and treatment of tachyarrhythmias in pediatric patients, *J Pediatr* 124:139-143, 1994.

Schamberger MS: Cardiac emergencies in children, *Pediatr Ann* 25:339-334, 1996.

24. Hyperkalemia

RICHARD BACHUR

OBJECTIVES

1. Manage hypovolemic shock.
2. Manage cardiopulmonary arrest.
3. Recognize and treat hyperkalemia.

Brief Presenting History

A 4-year-old male who has had bloody diarrhea for 3 days now has vomited 15 times over last 24 hours and has profound weakness.

Initial Vital Signs

P 160, BP 65/P, RR 40.
If asked: T 37.2° C, estimated weight 17 kg.

Initial Physical Examination

Profoundly pale, lethargic male, with grunting respirations.
- **Airway:** Patent.
- **Breathing:** Grunting, shallow respirations, lungs clear.
- **Circulation:** Tachycardic, no murmur, capillary refill time 3 to 4 seconds.
- Responds to voice appropriately, but no spontaneous speech.
- Abdomen with slight tenderness diffusely, liver edge at the right costal margin.
- Diarrhea tests heme positive.

Further History If Requested

- Weakness and vomiting have been progressive over last 24 hours.
- No urine output for 2 days.
- Intermittent confusion at home. May have had slight fever intermittently. No trauma or ingestion.
- Past medical history was unremarkable.
- No medications, NKDA, no history of travel.

Expected interventions	Complications

1. 100% O_2, assist with BVM.
   Cricoid pressure.
2. Monitors (ECG and pulse oximeter).
3. IV access attempt.
   Normal saline 20 ml/kg IV/IO.
4. Laboratory tests: Rapid glucose, ABG, CBC,
   electrolytes, type and cross, blood culture
   and stool culture, blood smear.
5. Call for **O-negative blood.**
	Vomits, requires suction.
	
	PIV unsuccessful. IO placement.

Progression

Patient is less responsive, more agitated. Capillary refill time is 4 to 5 seconds.
ECG monitor: Rate 140 with peaked T-waves.

Expected interventions	Complications

1. Rapid sequence intubation.
   Miller no. 2, 5.0 ETT.
   Atropine 0.02 mg/kg IV/IO.
   Midazolam 0.1 mg/kg IV/IO.
   Vecuronium 0.1 mg/kg IV/IO.
   Cricoid pressure.
   Place NG and end-tidal CO_2 monitor.
   Call for CXR to check ETT position.
2. Check pulses.
3. Repeat **normal saline** 20 ml/kg IV/IO
   or transfuse O-negative blood 10 ml/kg.
4. 12-Lead ECG.
5. Treat hyperkalemia.
   Hyperventilate.
   Calcium chloride 10 to 20 mg/kg IV/IO.
   Sodium bicarbonate 1 mEq/kg IV/IO.
   $D_{25}W$ 2 to 4 ml/kg, regular **insulin** 0.1 to
   0.2 unit/kg IV/IO.
   Kayexalate 1 g/kg PR.
   Albuterol 2.5 mg nebulizer.
6. Consider empiric antibiotics.
	If succinylcholine administered, cardiac arrest
	   and asystole develop.
	Vomits if cricoid pressure not applied.
	Right mainstem intubation.
	
	Pulses thready but palpable.

Progression

Asystole appears on the monitor. (See Appendix E, p. 218.)

Expected interventions	Complications
1. Check pulses.	No pulse.
2. Begin chest compressions.	
Check pulse.	Femoral pulse with compressions.
See Asystole (p. 198) in Chapter 4.	
3. **Epinephrine** 1:10,000, 0.1 ml/kg IV.	

Progression

Monitor reads sinus rhythm, rate 150.

Expected interventions	Complications
1. Check pulses.	Femoral pulse present.
2. Continue hyperkalemia therapy.	
3. Contact renal/dialysis service.	

Laboratory Results

Rapid glucose 80, ABG: pH 7.08, Pco_2 32, Po_2 190, HCO_3 6, Na 128, K 10.0, BUN 45, Cr 2.3, Hct 32.
Peripheral blood smear has evidence of hemolysis.

Additional Potential Complications

1. Patient presents with high-output cardiac failure and shock resulting from acute hemolysis. Aggressive fluid resuscitation pushes the patient into respiratory distress from worsening failure. Treatment includes **blood** transfusion and diuresis with **furosemide**.
2. Additional rhythms that may develop include idioventricular and ventricular fibrillation. Lack of response to an initial defibrillation attempt at 2 J/kg necessitates loading with **lidocaine** 1 mg/kg IV and repeating defibrillation at 4 J/kg.

Disposition

ICU, may require dialysis.

Discussion of Objectives

1. *Manage hypovolemic shock.*
   Hypovolemic shock in pediatric patients is treated initially with **isotonic crystalloid** at 20 ml/kg by rapid IV bolus. If reassessment reveals ongoing compromised perfusion, the 20 ml/kg bolus is repeated. Persistent hypovolemia despite isotonic crystalloid 40 ml/kg is treated with colloid 20 ml/kg IV such as **5% albumin**. Patients refractory to this aggressive therapy should be considered for unmatched **O-negative blood** in an acute situation followed by cross-matched blood as time allows, with close attention paid to ongoing losses.

Patients in septic shock receive aggressive volume resuscitation and may require vasopressors. *Note:* Aggressive fluid resuscitation leads to worsening shock if the patient has severe hemolysis and anemia and high-output cardiac failure. These patients are treated with cautious blood transfusion and **furosemide**.

2. *Manage cardiopulmonary arrest.*

   A team approach should be organized to simultaneously secure the airway (initially with BVM ventilation followed by endotracheal intubation), administer positive-pressure ventilation, and begin effective chest compressions. Pulses must be checked continuously during CPR by palpating the femoral or carotid artery. Medications should be administered in an algorithmic approach based on rhythm (see Cardiac Emergencies [p. 198] in Chapter 4). CPR should be continued until a pulse has been restored. Central access may be more helpful for delivery of medications.

3. *Recognize and treat hyperkalemia.*

   Recognition of hyperkalemia often requires suspicion based on the history, peaked T-waves on an ECG, or results of routine electrolyte studies. Besides peaked T-waves, slow idioventricular rhythms or wide complex rhythms should raise suspicion. Peaked T-waves frequently are not evident on typical cardiac monitors; a 12-lead ECG may be required.

   Treatment begins with administration of **calcium chloride** (preferred over gluconate, which requires a normally functioning liver to be metabolized) to stabilize cardiac muscle membranes. Potassium is driven into cells through alkalization, which is achieved by hyperventilation and the administration of **sodium bicarbonate**. **Insulin** and **glucose** therapy should also be considered to help move potassium into cells. **Kayexalate** 1 g/kg PR is given to bind potassium but may not be useful when gut ischemia is present.

Additional Comments

1. **Succinylcholine** is contraindicated in this situation (because of hyperkalemia) and would cause asystole (or idioventicular rhythm) immediately after administration. Other nondepolarizing paralytic agents such as **vecuronium** 0.1 to 0.2 mg/kg or **rocuronium** 0.1 to 1 mg/kg IV would be preferred.

2. Hyperkalemia in this scenario is due to renal failure caused by hemolytic uremic syndrome (HUS). Typical symptoms of HUS are bloody diarrhea and dehydration. Patients have a hemolytic anemia that may, in conjunction with bloody diarrhea, lead to significant anemia and hypertension. Renal failure is a potential complication of HUS that leads to hyperkalemia if left untreated.

REFERENCES

McClure RJ, Prasad VK, Brocklebank JT: Treatment of hyperkalaemia using intravenous and nebulised salbutamol, *Arch Dis Child* 70:126-128, 1994.

McDonald RA: Disorders of potassium balance, *Pediatr Ann* 24:31-37, 1995.

Quigley RP, Alexander SR: Acute renal failure. In Levin DL, Morriss FC, eds: *Essentials of pediatric intensive care*, St Louis, 1990, Quality Medical Publishing.

25. Cyanotic Spell

ANDREW ATZ

OBJECTIVES

1. Recognize the presentation of hypoxemia.
2. Understand the mechanism of cyanosis in tetralogy of Fallot.
3. Manage a cyanotic spell associated with tetralogy of Fallot.

Brief Presenting History

A 2-month-old female has a 24-hour history of vomiting, diarrhea, and a decrease in the usual number of wet diapers. Her father brought her in after she was unable to keep any formula down for the previous 6 hours.

Initial Vital Signs

P 170, BP 80/45, RR 50.
If asked: T 36.9° C (R), estimated weight 5 kg.
Pulse oximetry 93% in room air.

Initial Physical Examination

General appearance: Listless infant in father's arms.
If asked: Mucous membranes and lips dry. No skin tenting.
- **Airway:** Patent, good air movement.
- **Breathing:** Tachypneic with minimal intercostal retractions, clear, symmetric breath sounds.
- **Circulation:** Acyanotic, tachycardic, normal S_1 and S_2, III/VI systolic ejection murmur heard best at left upper sternal border, brachial and femoral pulses full.
- No hepatosplenomegaly.

Further History Given on Request

- Prenatal diagnosis by ultrasound of tetralogy of Fallot, asymptomatic to date.
- No medications.
- Last echocardiogram at 1 week of life: single "hole."
- Elective surgical repair planned at about 6 months of age.

Expected interventions	Complications
1. 100% Oxygen by face mask (proper fit). 2. Monitors (ECG, pulse oximeter). 3. IV access attempts.	Unable to start IV.

Progression

During IV attempts, patient becomes acutely irritable and cyanotic and murmur is no longer auscultated.

Repeat Vital Signs

P 180, RR 50, BP cannot be measured despite good pulses, pulse oximeter 65%.

Expected Interventions

First-line therapy without drugs:
1. "Deintensify" the room. Let the parent hold and comfort the child.
2. Knee-chest position (may irritate this already anxious child).
3. Oxygen as tolerated.

Progression

Patient becomes more irritable and persistently cyanotic, pulse oximeter in low 40s. All efforts to calm the infant and end the cyanotic spell fail.

Expected interventions	Complications
Secondary therapy, initial drug management 1. **Morphine** 0.1 to 0.2 mg/kg SQ. 2. 100% Oxygen. 3. IV access attempt. **Normal saline** 10 to 20 ml/kg IV/IO. 4. Contact cardiology department.	 If IV unsuccessful, place IO.

Progression

Option 1: Initial drug management is successful. Patient regains color and pulse oximeter is now 97% with blow-by O_2.

Option 2: Initial drug management is successful, but only temporarily. Patient reverts to cyanotic state.

Option 3: Initial drug management fails. Patient becomes profoundly cyanotic.

Expected interventions	Complications

Option 1

1. Continue low-stress environment.

Patient reverts to cyanotic state if stressed.

Option 2

1. Repeat **morphine** 0.1 to 0.2 mg/kg IV/IO/SQ.

Patient becomes apneic.

2. BVM-assisted ventilations.
3. Rapid sequence intubation.
   Miller no. 1 blade, 3.5 to 4.0 ETT.
   Atropine 0.01 mg/kg IV.
   +/−**Midazolam** 0.1 mg/kg IV.
   Vecuronium 0.1 to 0.2 mg/kg IV.
   Cricoid pressure.
   Place NG and end-tidal CO_2 monitor.
   CXR for ETT position.
4. If cyanosis persists:
   Phenylephrine 0.1 mg/kg IV/IO bolus
       2 to 10 µg/kg/min continuous infusion or
       methoxamine 0.1 mg/kg IV.

If narcotic effect is allowed to abate without intubation, patient awakes and is acutely cyanotic.

Vomits if no cricoid pressure.

Option 3

1. Aggressive vasoconstrictor therapy.
   Phenylephrine 0.1 mg/kg IV bolus 2 to 10
       µg/kg/min continuous infusion or
       methoxamine 0.1 mg/kg IV.
2. Consider **sodium bicarbonate** 0.5 mEq/kg IV.
3. Rapid sequence intubation.
   Miller no. 1 blade, 3.5 to 4.0 ETT.
   Atropine 0.01 mg/kg IV.
   +/−**Midazolam** 0.1 mg/kg IV.
   Vecuronium 0.1 to 0.2 mg/kg IV.
   Cricoid pressure.
   Place NG and end-tidal CO_2 monitor.
   CXR for ETT position.
4. Contact cardiac surgery department.

If narcotic effect is allowed to abate without intubation, patient awakes and is acutely cyanotic.

Vomits if no cricoid pressure.

Profound hypoxia despite full medical management therapies.

Disposition

Option 1: Cardiac floor versus ICU for close cardiac monitoring.

Option 2: ICU for close cardiac monitoring, paralysis, and sedation. The patient will require a palliative Blalock-Taussig (subclavian to pulmonary artery) shunt or complete surgical repair when her condition stabilizes.

Option 3: Surgical emergency. While awaiting OR, continue phenylephrine continuous IV infusion to maximize systemic vascular resistance.

Additional Potential Complications

1. This scenario may be made more difficult by not offering the history of congenital heart disease. The infant has cyanosis and cardiac murmur, and the team is required to make the proper diagnosis and institute therapy.

Discussion of Objectives

1. *Recognize the presentation of hypoxemia.*

   Hypoxemia in an infant may not always be readily recognized by the physical examination alone. Hypoxemic infants need not be overtly cyanotic. They may have nonspecific symptoms such as fussiness or poor feeding. Pulse oximetry is a rapid, noninvasive method of confirming hypoxemia except in patients with anemia or hemoglobin bound by molecules other than oxygen (i.e., carbon monoxide, methemoglobinemia).

   Episodic hypoxemia and hypercyanotic spells must be expected in infants with tetralogy of Fallot.

2. *Understand the mechanism of cyanosis in tetralogy of Fallot.*

   Tetralogy of Fallot consists of four structural cardiac abnormalities: ventricular septal defect (VSD), right ventricular hypertrophy (RVH), right ventricular outflow tract stenosis, and dextroposition of the aorta. Cyanosis results from decreased pulmonary blood flow and right-to-left shunting of deoxygenated blood through the VSD to the systemic circulation.

   Hypercyanotic spells in tetralogy of Fallot occur during periods of dehydration, on waking from prolonged sleep, and during periods of acute agitation such as invasive procedures. The pathophysiology of these events relates to changes in cardiac output and venous blood return to the heart, as well as changes in systemic vascular resistance (SVR).

   Loss of a right ventricular outflow tract murmur that had been previously auscultated indicates dramatic decrease in pulmonary blood flow.

3. *Manage a cyanotic spell associated with tetralogy of Fallot.*

   Treatment of a "tet" spell begins with attempts to console and position the patient. Every attempt is made to calm the patient. Parents are generally best at consoling a frantic infant. All aggressive treatments of spells (e.g., IV attempts) can actually exacerbate hypoxemia. Knee-chest position often helps reverse right-to-left blood flow and cyanosis by increasing SVR.

   If positioning and calming fail, oxygen and **morphine sulfate** should be administered. Oxygen offers small improvement in most cases but may not provide improvement in episodes of severely compromised pulmonary blood flow. The dose of **morphine** is 0.1 to 0.2 mg/kg SQ if no IV access exists. The mechanism of morphine in hypercyanotic spells is not fully understood. IV fluids can be given to provide adequate right ventricular volume, especially in patients with dehydration. For acidotic patients, **sodium bicarbonate** should be administered. In severely hypoxic patients resistant to the above therapies, aggressive vasoconstrictor therapy is initiated and rapid sequence intubation provided when indicated. Vasopressors such as **phenylephrine** and **methoxamine** acutely raise the SVR. Continuous IV infusion may be required.

A hypercyanotic spell that cannot be ended is a surgical emergency. The cardiology and surgery departments should be involved early.

REFERENCES

Adams FH, Emmanouilides GC, Riemenschneider TA, eds: *Moss' heart disease in infants, children, and adolescents*, ed 4, Baltimore, 1989, Williams & Wilkins, pp 273-288.

Fyler DC, ed: *Nadas' pediatric cardiology*, Philadelphia, 1992, Hanley & Belfus, pp 471-491.

Gewitz MH, Vetter VL: Cardiac emergencies. In Fleisher GR, Ludwig S, eds: *Textbook of pediatric emergency medicine*, ed 3, Baltimore, 1993, Williams & Wilkins, pp 567-569.

TRAUMA
26. Closed Head Injury

MARK G. ROBACK

OBJECTIVES

1. Recognize mechanisms for multiple blunt trauma, and be aware that resuscitation begins with the ABCs.
2. Aggressively treat hypovolemic shock with fluid resuscitation.
3. Manage closed head injury.

Brief Presenting History

Pedestrian versus auto. A 5-year-old male has been struck by a car. The child's father picked him up and brought him in directly to be seen.

Initial Vital Signs

P 110, BP 110/70, RR 24.
If asked: T 36.2° C (R), estimated weight 20 kg.

Initial Physical Examination

General appearance: Moaning, verbal but confused.
If asked: Eyes open in response to speech, ecchymotic swelling over left frontal region.
- **Airway:** Patent.
- **Breathing:** Breath sounds full and clear bilaterally, slight tachypnea.
- **Circulation:** Heart tones normal, capillary refill time 2 to 3 seconds, pulses full.
- Obeys commands (GCS 13), pupils equal in size and reactive.
- Abdomen soft but tender LUQ with large ecchymosis on left flank and hip.
- Pelvis nontender to palpation, no crepitus or instability noted.
- Rectal with normal tone, heme negative, prostate normal.
- Genitalia atraumatic.
- Moves all extremities, no deformities.

Further History Given on Request

Patient ran into the street and was struck by a car moving at 20 to 30 mph. He was thrown 10 to 15 feet, striking his head on the pavement after landing on his left hip and side.

Expected interventions	Complications
1. 100% O_2, C-spine immobilization/backboard. 2. Monitors (ECG and oximeter). 3. Two large-bore IVs, placed with **normal saline/Ringer's lactate** 20 ml/kg IV. Call for **O-negative blood**. 4. Laboratory tests: Rapid glucose, type and cross, CBC, ABG, amylase/lipase. 5. Radiology department called for chest, pelvis, lateral neck x-rays. 6. Surgery and neurosurgery departments called. 7. UA, temperature.	If difficulty starting IV, then IO placement. Vomiting requires suction and log roll.

Initial Laboratory Findings

Hct 33, ABG: pH 7.38, Pco_2 38, Po_2 240, rapid glucose 90.

Repeat Vital Signs

P 150, BP 90/40, RR 30, capillary refill time 3 to 4 seconds.

Progression

Respiratory effort decreases.

Expected interventions	Complications
1. 100% O_2, BVM-assisted ventilation applied. 2. Prepare for rapid sequence intubation.	Vomits if no cricoid pressure.

Radiographs

CXR negative, pelvis negative, C-spine (lateral) clear.

Progression

Patient becomes poorly responsive.

Expected interventions	Complications
1. Place IO if no IV access. Repeat **normal saline/Ringer's lactate** 20 ml/kg IV.	Patient vomits, requiring suctioning after log roll.

2. Rapid sequence intubation.
   Miller no. 2 blade, 5.5 ETT.
   Atropine 0.02 mg/kg IV/IO.
   Lidocaine 1 mg/kg IV/IO.
   Midazolam 0.1 mg/kg IV/IO.
   Vecuronium 0.1 to 0.2 mg/kg IV/IO or
   Rocuronium 0.6 to 1 mg/kg IV/IO or
   Succinylcholine 1 mg/kg IV/IO after defasciculating **vecuronium** 0.01 mg/kg IV/IO.
   Cricoid pressure.
   Place NG and end-tidal CO_2 monitor.
   CXR for ETT position.
	Right mainstem intubation.
	
	Tube falls out if not properly taped and cared for.
	
	Vomits if no cricoid pressure or no NG tube placed.

3. Hyperventilate (P_{CO_2} 30 to 35).	
4. Place central venous line (CVL).	
5. Place Foley catheter.	

Progression

After paralytic wears off, patient has a generalized tonic-clonic seizure.

Expected interventions	Complications
1. **Lorazepam** 0.05 to 0.1 mg/kg IV/IO.	Persistent seizure.
2. Repeat **lorazepam** 0.1 mg/kg IV/IO. Load with **phenytoin** 10 to 20 mg/kg IV/IO over 20 minutes.	Cardiovascular collapse if phenytoin given as IV push.
3. **Pancuronium** 0.1 mg/kg IV.	

Progression

Capillary refill time 3 to 4 seconds, HR 170, BP 70/35.

Expected Interventions

1. Give **O-negative blood** 20 ml/kg IV.
2. Consider diagnostic peritoneal lavage (DPL). See comments on DPL below.

Additional Potential Complications

1. Development of dyspnea with unilateral decrease in breath sounds and desaturation indicative of a pneumothorax or hemothorax requiring emergency chest tube placement.
2. Development of hematuria, an indication for renal/GU workup.

Disposition

If hemodynamically stable after fluid resuscitation, CT scanner for CT of head and abdomen.

Discussion of Objectives

1. *Recognize mechanisms for multiple blunt trauma, and be aware that resuscitation begins with the ABCs.*

   A pedestrian struck by a moving vehicle is a mechanism associated with major traumatic injuries. Resuscitation begins with the primary survey of the ABCs. Assessment and control of the **airway** with attention to cervical spine immobilization are first, followed by administration of 100% oxygen as **breathing** is evaluated and treated. **Circulation** is assessed, two large-bore IVs are placed, and fluid resuscitation is begun. After a rapid neurologic examination the patient is exposed so that all injuries may be evaluated. After this resuscitation phase the patient is examined completely in the secondary survey. During the definitive care phase all injuries are addressed. The trauma surgeons, orthopedists, and neurosurgeons are responsible for the definitive care phase of trauma. See Cervical Spine Immobilization (p. 11) in Chapter 2 and Trauma (p. 203) in Chapter 4.

2. *Aggressively treat hypovolemic shock with fluid resuscitation.*

   Initial fluid resuscitation consists of **isotonic crystalloid** 20 ml/kg given rapidly and repeated if reassessment reveals continued shock based on tachycardia and poor perfusion. Low blood pressure is a late finding of shock in pediatric patients because of compensatory mechanisms. If patients display tachycardia, diminished pulses, prolonged capillary refill time, or cool mottled skin, hypovolemia is likely; aggressive fluid resuscitation should be started.

   Colloid should be added if hypotension persists after administration of isotonic crystalloid 40 ml/kg. Type **O-negative whole blood** should be used if cross-matched, type-specific whole blood is not available.

   Sites of ongoing blood loss must be investigated. The chest, abdomen, retroperitoneum, and pelvis are areas of "silent" bleeding that require evaluation by physical examination and CT scan. Long bone fractures, especially those involving the femurs, can lead to significant bleeding.

   Intracranial bleeding typically does not lead to overt hypotension, since the cranial vault allows only a finite amount of blood loss. However, in infants with open sutures growth of the intracranial space is possible and large amounts of blood may accumulate.

   Vasopressors, steroids, and sodium bicarbonate have no role in the initial management of hypovolemic shock in trauma. The 3:1 rule should be kept in mind; patients require 300 ml of crystalloid for each 100 ml of blood lost.

3. *Manage closed head injury.*

   For a GCS of 8 or less (see Appendix F, p. 220).

   a. Rapid sequence intubation.

   Atropine 0.02 mg/kg IV.

Lidocaine 1 mg/kg IV.

Midazolam 0.1 to 0.3 mg/kg IV.

   Thiopental may exacerbate hypotension and should not be used in this case.

Vecuronium 0.1 to 0.2 mg/kg IV or **rocuronium** 0.6 to 1 mg/kg IV.

   Succinylcholine may result in ICP elevation but is not absolutely contraindicated in head injuries. A defasciculating dose of **vecuronium** 0.01 mg/kg IV is given before succinyl-choline. Succinylcholine is contraindicated in crush injuries, severe burns (hyperkalemia), glaucoma (increased ocular pressure), penetrating eye injuries, and significant neuromuscular disease. (See Rapid Sequence Intubation [p. 10] in Chapter 2.)

   b. Hyperventilation. Patients are hyperventilated to decrease intracranial pressure, with a P_{CO_2} goal of approximately 30 to 35.

   c. **Mannitol** 0.5 to 1 g/kg IV as an osmotic diuretic (use is contraindicated in hypotension).

In the management of a patient with increased intracranial pressure the goal is to maintain cerebral perfusion pressure (CPP):

$$CPP \ = \ MAP \ - \ ICP \ (MAP \ = \ \text{mean arterial pressure; } ICP \ = \ \text{intracranial pressure})$$

Thus volume resuscitation with maintenance of mean arterial pressure is vital. See Increased Intracranial Pressure (p. 196) in Chapter 4.

Additional Comments

1. Early notification of the surgical trauma team and neurosurgery department is essential.
2. Physical examination points to be stressed include:
   a. Proper evaluation of the pelvis.
   b. Examination of the rectum and genitalia before Foley catheter placement, which is contraindicated in the presence of an overriding prostate, blood at the urethral meatus, or blood in the scrotum.
   c. Examination of the entire patient, including the back.
3. ABG: In a patient with altered mental status and multiple trauma, early assessment for hypoxia and secondary metabolic acidosis.
4. Procedures (if indicated; see Chapter 2):
   a. Femoral CVL.
   b. Chest tube.
5. Call the blood bank for **whole blood, packed red blood cells (PRBCs), or O-negative blood** if necessary (whatever is available immediately), early in the resuscitation effort.
6. If evidence of midfacial trauma is present, an oral-gastric (OG) tube should be placed rather than a nasogastric tube (NG) because of potential facial bone (cribriform plate) fractures.
7. Diagnostic peritoneal lavage (DPL). Used in trauma to evaluate the peritoneal cavity for bleeding, the DPL is seldom used in pediatrics because most causes of pediatric intraperitoneal bleeding such as liver and splenic lacerations are now managed without surgery. One potential indication is the hypotensive pediatric patient with head and abdominal injuries. If the DPL is negative, the patient may be sent to the CT scanner to evaluate for head injury. A positive DPL would lead to immediate exploratory laparotomy.

REFERENCES

Committee on Trauma, American College of Surgeons: *Advanced trauma life support, 1988 reference manual*, Chicago, 1988, American College of Surgeons.

Dolan M: Head trauma. In Barkin RM: *Pediatric emergency medicine: concepts and clinical practice*, ed 2, St Louis, 1997, Mosby.

Kaufman BA, Dacey RG: Acute management of closed head injury in childhood, *Pediatr Ann* 23:18-28, 1994.

Manary MJ, Jaffe DM: Cervical spine injuries in children, *Pediatr Ann* 25:423-428, 1996.

Ziegler MM, Templeton JM: Major trauma. In Fleisher GR, Ludwig S, ed: *Textbook of pediatric emergency medicine*, ed 3, Baltimore, 1993, Williams & Wilkins, pp 1089-1102.

27. Blunt Abdominal Trauma

GLENN FARIES AND MARK G. ROBACK

OBJECTIVES

1. Recognize mechanisms for multiple blunt trauma, and be aware that resuscitation begins with the ABCs.
2. Aggressively manage hypovolemic shock with fluid resuscitation.
3. Formulate the differential diagnosis of shock in blunt abdominal trauma.
4. Identify and manage blunt abdominal trauma.

Brief Presenting History

A 7-year-old male riding a bicycle collided with a slow-moving car. The bicycle hit the front end of the car, and the child was thrown up onto the hood of the vehicle.

Initial Vital Signs

HR 158, RR 45, BP 100/65.
If asked: T 36.8° C (R), estimated weight 25 kg.

Initial Physical Examination

General appearance: Alert, conversing appropriately but anxious and pale, mild respiratory distress.
If asked:
- **Airway:** Patent, normal speech.
- **Breathing:** Mild tachypnea, clear to auscultation, no bruises over chest or tenderness to palpation.
- **Circulation:** Tachycardic, pale, clammy, cool, capillary refill time 3 to 4 seconds.
- Pupils equal and reactive, extraocular movements intact, fundoscopy normal, no hemotympanum.
- No evident head trauma, neck nontender.
- Neurologic: Moves all extremities on command, tone normal, strength bilaterally equal.
- Abdomen: Distended, paucity of bowel sounds, contusion in epigastric area and left upper quadrant, diffusely tender.
- Rectal: Normal tone, heme negative, prostate normal.
- Genitourinary: Testes normal, no blood at urethral meatus.
- Pelvis: Stable, back nontender.
- Extremities: Superficial abrasions to palms, knees, and left shoulder.

Further History Given on Request

- The child was wearing a helmet, found in two pieces at the scene.
- No loss of consciousness. The handlebars struck the child's abdomen.
- Past medical history: Negative, NKDA.

Expected interventions	Complications
1. 100% O_2, nonrebreather. Immobilize cervical spine.	Vomits; log roll and suction.
2. Monitors (ECG and pulse oximeter).	
3. Two large-bore IVs. **Normal saline** 20 ml/kg IV.	IV attempt unsuccessful, necessitating CVL attempt.
4. Laboratory tests: CBC, type and cross, amylase, UA.	
5. Radiology: CXR, lateral neck, pelvis film.	

Repeat Vital Signs

HR 176, RR 60, BP 80/35, pulse oximetry 92%.

Progression

Patient becomes paler, more diaphoretic, and less alert. Rapid shallow breathing, occasional grunting respirations. The abdomen is becoming increasingly distended.

Expected interventions	Complications
1. Repeat bolus of **normal saline** 20 ml/kg IV. Call blood bank for O-negative blood.	IV infiltrates.
2. BVM-assisted ventilation. Prepare for rapid sequence intubation.	

Progression

Patient becomes combative and intermittently unresponsive with minimal respiratory effort.

Expected interventions	Complications
1. Rapid sequence intubation. Consider: **Atropine** 0.02 mg/kg IV. **Midazolam** 0.1 mg/kg IV. **Vecuronium** 0.1 to 0.2 mg/kg IV or **rocuronium** 0.6 to 1 mg/kg IV or **succinylcholine** 1 mg/kg IV after defasciculating **vecuronium** 0.01 mg/kg IV. Cricoid pressure. Place NG and end-tidal CO_2 monitor. CXR for ETT position.	Right mainstem intubation. Tube falls out if not properly taped and cared for. Vomits if no cricoid pressure or NG tube placed.
2. **O-negative blood** 20 ml/kg IV.	
3. Foley catheter.	

Additional Potential Complications

1. Overzealous bagging leads to pneumothorax.
2. Failure to recognize need for aggressive fluid resuscitation leads to pulseless electrical activity (PEA).

Disposition

OR for exploration if unable to achieve hemodynamic stability. If patient is stable, radiology department for CT scan of the abdomen.

Discussion of Objectives

1. *Recognize mechanisms for multiple blunt trauma, and be aware that resuscitation begins with the ABCs.*

   Bicycle injuries represent mechanisms that may be associated with major traumatic injuries. Resuscitation begins with the primary survey of the ABCs. Assessment and control of the **airway** with attention to cervical spine immobilization are first. The patient is given 100% oxygen as **breathing** is evaluated. **Circulation** is assessed, two large-bore IVs are placed, and fluid resuscitation is begun. After a rapid neurologic examination the patient is exposed so that all injuries may be evaluated. All problems identified in the primary survey are addressed in the resuscitation phase. In the secondary survey the patient is completely examined and other problems are identified.

   During the definitive care phase all injuries are addressed. The trauma surgeons, orthopedic surgeons, and neurosurgeons are responsible for the definitive care phase of trauma. (See Cervical Spine Immobilization [p. 11] in Chapter 2 and Trauma [p. 203] in Chapter 4.)

2. *Aggressively manage hypovolemic shock with fluid resuscitation.*

   Initial fluid resuscitation consists of **isotonic crystalloid** 20 ml/kg given rapidly and repeated if reassessment reveals ongoing losses or hypotension resulting from tachycardia and poor perfusion. In pediatric patients low blood pressure is a late finding of shock because of compensatory mechanisms. If patients display tachycardia, diminished pulses, prolonged capillary refill time, or cool mottled skin, hypovolemia must be considered and aggressive fluid resuscitation begun. Persistent hypotension despite isotonic crystalloid 40 ml/kg requires the addition of colloid. Type **O-negative whole blood** is used if cross-matched, type-specific whole blood is not available.

   Sites of ongoing blood loss must be investigated. The abdomen, retroperitoneum, and pelvis are areas of "silent" bleeding that require evaluation by physical examination and CT scan. Long bone fractures, especially those involving the femurs, can lead to significant bleeding.

   Intracranial bleeding typically does not lead to overt hypotension because the cranial vault allows only a finite amount of blood loss. However, in infants with open sutures the intracranial space may grow and large amounts of blood may accumulate.

   Vasopressors, steroids, and sodium bicarbonate have no role in the initial management of hypovolemic shock in trauma. The "3:1 rule" applies; patients require 300 ml of crystalloid for each 100 ml of blood lost.

3. *Formulate the differential diagnosis of shock in blunt abdominal trauma.*

   Blunt abdominal trauma (BAT) may cause bleeding and hypovolemic shock from several sources. The workup of bleeding caused by BAT must include investigation of the peritoneal cavity, retroperitoneum, and pelvis.

Lacerations of the liver and spleen are common causes of peritoneal bleeding. Bowel disruption and mesenteric bleeding are also important causes of peritoneal blood loss.

Retroperitoneal bleeding may be significant and must be considered because bleeding at this site is usually not obvious on physical examination. Retroperitoneal sites include the kidneys, adrenal glands, and bladder. Another "silent" area of bleeding is the pelvis, which emphasizes the importance of the pelvic film. Fractures of the pelvic skeleton may lead to massive blood loss into the pelvis.

Abdominal injuries caused by bicycle handlebars are common in pediatrics. Injuries to be considered include lacerations of the pancreas, liver, and spleen. Duodenal hematomas may also occur. Difficult to diagnose and often not visualized by abdominal CT, duodenal hematomas should be suspected in patients with persistent tenderness and signs or symptoms of obstruction such as vomiting.

The use of lap-belt restraint without shoulder harness results in a series of injuries referred to as the lap-belt complex. Sudden flexion of the child's torso around a fixed lap belt may lead to intraabdominal injuries of hollow viscera and the pancreas and compression injuries of the lower thoracic and lumbar spine.

4. *Identify and manage blunt abdominal trauma.*

The management of BAT begins with attention to the ABCs, including emphasis on aggressive volume resuscitation as discussed previously. Evaluation of the hematocrit offers information about amount of bleeding but may not show a significant decline initially. Urinalysis is performed to investigate possible renal trauma. Blood in the urine is a nonspecific marker for significant abdominal trauma that does not necessarily involve the kidneys. An elevated amylase level is indicative of pancreatic trauma, but the concentration may be high with injuries to the salivary glands and also may not be elevated initially. The CT scan of the abdomen remains the gold standard for investigating BAT in pediatric patients. Limitations include evaluation of the duodenum for hematoma and the hemodynamically unstable patient who requires emergency operative evaluation.

Diagnostic peritoneal lavage (DPL) is used in adult BAT to assess the peritoneal cavity for bleeding. Indications for DPL in the pediatric population are limited because most causes of pediatric intraperitoneal bleeding such as liver and spleen lacerations are now managed nonoperatively. One potential indication is the hypotensive pediatric patient with head and abdominal injuries. A positive DPL would lead to immediate exploratory laparotomy. If the DPL is negative, the patient may be sent for CT scanning to evaluate the head while receiving further volume resuscitation.

Studies are under way to evaluate emergency diagnostic abdominal ultrasound as a means of ascertaining whether significant intraabdominal fluid (blood) is present. Its use in adult centers is becoming widespread, but it is not yet used widely in children.

The cornerstone of management of BAT is adequate volume resuscitation as discussed previously and aggressive diagnostic evaluation of potential causes of shock. Much of pediatric BAT is managed nonoperatively, but surgical intervention may be lifesaving in patients with ongoing blood loss.

Additional Comments

1. Early notification of the surgical trauma team and neurosurgery department is essential.
2. Points to be stressed in the physical examination include:
   a. Proper evaluation of the pelvis.
   b. Examination of the rectum and genitalia before Foley catheter placement, which is contraindicated in the presence of an overriding prostate, blood at the urethral meatus, or blood in the scrotum.
   c. Examination of the entire patient, including the back.
3. ABG: In a patient with altered mental status and multiple trauma, early assessment for hypoxia and secondary metabolic acidosis.
4. Procedures (if indicated; see Chapter 2):
   a. Femoral CVL.
   b. Chest thoracostomy tube.
5. Call the blood bank for **whole blood**, **packed red blood cells**, or **O-negative blood** if necessary (whatever is available immediately) early in the resuscitation effort.
6. Respiratory compromise can result from shock or abdominal distention in patients with no pulmonary or cardiac injuries.

REFERENCES

Committee on Trauma, American College of Surgeons: *Advanced trauma life support, 1988 core course reference manual*, Chicago, 1988, American College of Surgeons.

Foltin GL, Cooper A: Abdominal trauma. In Barkin RM: *Pediatric emergency medicine: concepts and clinical practice*, ed 2, St Louis, 1997, Mosby.

Jaffe D, Wesson D: Emergency management of blunt trauma in children, *N Engl J Med* 324:1477-1482, 1991.

Nordenholz KE et al: Ultrasound in the evaluation and management of blunt abdominal trauma, *Ann Emerg Med* 29:357-366, 1997.

Saladino RA, Lund DP: Abdominal trauma. In Fleisher GR, Ludwig S, eds: *Textbook of pediatric emergency medicine*, ed 3, Baltimore, 1993, Williams & Wilkins, pp 1167-1174.

28. Blunt Thoracic Trauma

MARK G. ROBACK

OBJECTIVES

1. Recognize mechanisms for multiple blunt trauma, and be aware that resuscitation begins with the ABCs.
2. Aggressively manage hypovolemic shock with fluid resuscitation.
3. Formulate the differential diagnosis of respiratory distress in blunt thoracic trauma.
4. Identify and manage blunt thoracic trauma.

Brief Presenting History

A 16-year-old male driver has been in a head-on collision with another vehicle at approximately 30 mph. The patient complains of pain on the right side.

Initial Vital Signs

HR 135, RR 40, BP 110/70.
If asked: T 37.4° C (R), estimated weight 70 kg.

Initial Physical Examination

General appearance: Alert, diaphoretic and pale, tachypneic.
If asked:

- **Airway:** Patent, patient is able to speak.
- **Breathing:** Obvious dyspnea, large ecchymosis over right chest, decreased breath sounds on right, no tracheal deviation.
- **Circulation:** Heart rate regular, heart tones not displaced, capillary refill time 3 to 4 seconds.
- Pupils equal and reactive, extraocular movements intact, disc margins sharp.
- No obvious head trauma, neck supple, nontender to palpation.
- Abdomen not distended, positive bowel sounds, tender right upper quadrant.
- Rectal tone normal, heme negative.
- Pelvis intact, back atraumatic.
- Neurologic: Alert, follows commands.
- Extremities: No obvious deformities, moves all extremities equally.

Further History Given on Request

Unrestrained driver, chest struck steering wheel.

- No loss of consciousness, he did not strike his head.
- No ejection or roll-over; driver of the other vehicle dead at the scene.
- Previous medical history: Negative.
- No medications, NKDA.

Expected interventions	Complications
1. 100% O_2 by nonrebreather. Immobilize cervical spine and trunk. 2. Monitors (ECG and oximeter). 3. Two large-bore IVs. **Normal saline** 20 ml/kg IV. 4. Laboratory tests: ABG, type and cross, CBC, amylase. 5. Call blood bank for **O-negative blood**. 6. Call for CXR, pelvis and lateral neck x-rays.	Vomiting, necessitating suction and log roll. IV access unsuccessful, necessitating femoral CVL.

Repeat Vital Signs

Pulse oximeter 82% in room air, HR 150, RR 45, BP 100/60.

Laboratory Results

ABG: pH 7.3, P_{CO_2} 49, P_{O_2} 90, spun Hct 34.

Progression

Acutely more dyspneic, desaturation despite 100% O_2 by nonrebreather.

Repeat Vital Signs

HR 75, RR 8, BP 95/55.

Expected interventions	Complications
1. Thoracentesis in right side of chest with 20-gauge needle. 2. Prepare for rapid sequence intubation. 3. Repeat **normal saline** 20 ml/kg IV. See Thoracentesis (p. 12) and Thoracostomy Tube (p. 13) in Chapter 2.	No thoracentesis or chest tube results in respiratory arrest and asystole.

Progression

Needle thoracostomy results in large rush of air, but the patient now has agonal respirations, persistent hypoxia, and hypotension. RR 6, BP 80/P, pulse oximetry 87%.

Expected interventions	Complications

1. Rapid sequence intubation.
    7.5 cuffed ETT.
    Mac/Miller no. 3 blade.
    Midazolam 0.1 mg/kg IV.
    Vecuronium 0.1 to 0.2 mg/kg IV or
        rocuronium 0.6 to 1 mg/kg IV or
        succinylcholine 1 mg/kg IV after
        defasciculating **vecuronium** 0.01 mg/kg IV.
    Cricoid pressure.
    Place NG and end-tidal CO_2 monitor.
2. Place thoracostomy tube (34 to 36 Fr).
 	
3. Call for CXR.
4. Repeat **normal saline** 20 ml/kg IV.
5. Repeat ABG and Hct.
See Thoracostomy Tube (p. 13) in Chapter 2.
	Right mainstem intubation results in ineffective ventilation.
	Tube falls out if not properly taped and cared for.
	
	Vomits if no cricoid pressure or NG tube placed.
	Chest tube placed inferior to rib, resulting in chest wall bleeding.
	
	Failure to fluid resuscitate aggressively results in hypotension and asystole.

Progression

Chest tube produces 250 ml of blood, BP is 70/P.

Expected Interventions

1. **O-negative blood** 20 ml/kg.

Additional Potential Complications

1. Rather than hemothorax or pneumothorax, respiratory distress is due to flail chest, necessitating early intubation and positive-pressure ventilation.
2. Head injury with altered mental status in addition to chest trauma.
3. Cardiac tamponade caused by pericardial bleeding, resulting in pulseless electrical activity (PEA) that requires pericardiocentesis.

Disposition

When hemodynamically stable, to radiology department for CT of the abdomen. If persistent bloody chest tube output, OR for thoracotomy.

Discussion of Objectives

1. *Recognize mechanisms for multiple blunt trauma, and be aware that resuscitation begins with the ABCs.*
   Motor vehicle collisions represent mechanisms associated with major traumatic injuries. Resuscitation begins with the primary survey of the ABCs. Assessment and control of the **air-**

way with attention to cervical spine immobilization are first. The patient is given 100% oxygen as **breathing** is evaluated. **Circulation** is assessed, two large-bore IVs are placed, and fluid resuscitation is begun. After a rapid neurologic examination the patient is exposed so that all injuries may be evaluated. All problems identified in the primary survey are addressed in the resuscitation phase. In the secondary survey the patient is completely examined and other problems are identified.

During the definitive care phase all injuries are addressed. The trauma surgeons, orthopedic surgeons, and neurosurgeons are responsible for the definitive care phase of trauma. See Cervical Spine Immobilization (p. 11) in Chapter 2 and Trauma (p. 203) in Chapter 4.

2. *Aggressively manage hypovolemic shock with fluid resuscitation.*

Initial fluid resuscitation consists of **isotonic crystalloid** 20 ml/kg given rapidly and repeated if reassessment reveals ongoing losses or hypotension resulting from tachycardia and poor perfusion. In pediatric patients low blood pressure is a late finding of shock because of compensatory mechanisms. If patients display tachycardia, diminished pulses, prolonged capillary refill time, or cool mottled skin, hypovolemia must be considered and aggressive fluid resuscitation begun. Persistent hypotension despite isotonic crystalloid 40 ml/kg requires the addition of colloid. Type **O-negative whole blood** is used if cross-matched, type-specific whole blood is not available.

Sites of ongoing blood loss must be investigated. The abdomen, retroperitoneum, and pelvis are areas of "silent" bleeding that require evaluation by physical examination and CT scan. Long bone fractures, especially those involving the femurs, can lead to significant bleeding.

Intracranial bleeding typically does not lead to overt hypotension because the cranial vault allows only a finite amount of blood loss. However, in infants with open sutures the intracranial space may grow and large amounts of blood may accumulate.

Vasopressors, steroids, and sodium bicarbonate have no role in the initial management of hypovolemic shock in trauma. The "3:1" rule should be kept in mind; patients require 300 ml of crystalloid for each 100 ml of blood lost.

3. *Formulate the differential diagnosis of respiratory distress in blunt thoracic trauma.*

Respiratory distress in blunt chest trauma may result from one or more of the following: simple pneumothorax, tension pneumothorax, hemothorax, pulmonary contusion, cardiac tamponade or contusion, flail chest, or aortic or tracheal/bronchial disruption. Extrathoracic causes of tachypnea and respiratory distress include significant abdominal distention from gastric air or intraabdominal blood.

Tension pneumothorax should be suspected in patients with respiratory distress and unilateral chest findings. Decreased breath sounds, deviation of the trachea or heart sounds, and hyperresonance to percussion suggest the presence of air in the pleural cavity. Dullness to percussion may be elicited in patients with hemothorax.

Injuries to the thoracic aorta and great vessels must be suspected in injuries involving great force such as motor vehicle collisions or falls from great heights. Fractures of the first or second ribs or scapula suggest that significant force was involved and are an indicator for injury to the great vessels. CXR findings to recognize include widening of the mediastinum, blurring of the aortic knob, and depression of the left mainstem bronchus.

Paradoxical chest wall movement leading to ineffective ventilation is the result of flail chest injuries. Fractures to adjacent ribs or multiple ribs lead to separation of a portion of the chest from the thorax. During inspiration the flail segment moves independent of the chest, resulting in severe respiratory distress that requires positive-pressure ventilation.

Flail chest is relatively uncommon in children because of the elasticity of the chest wall. Typically, massive force is involved, leading to a high incidence of associated injuries such as pulmonary contusion, hemothorax, pneumothorax, and injury to the heart and great vessels or trachea and bronchial tree.

4. *Identify and manage blunt thoracic trauma.*

The presence of unilateral decreased breath sounds suggests pneumothorax, hemothorax, or hemopneumothorax. When desaturation occurs despite maximal oxygen delivery, or hypotension despite aggressive fluid resuscitation, surgical or needle aspiration of the chest is indicated. In this case there is no time for confirmation of diagnosis by chest radiograph. Deviation of the trachea or cardiac sounds should be sought as evidence of a tension pneumothorax. Needle thoracentesis should be performed by means of a large-bore IV catheter connected to a three-way stopcock and 60 ml syringe. The needle should be inserted into the thoracic cavity over the second rib in the midclavicular line.

After palliation by needle thoracentesis a chest tube is placed over the fourth rib in the midaxillary line. If no improvement is seen, the tube is redirected posteriorly in an attempt to remove blood. Needling the chest may not be sufficient to extract blood; a chest tube should be placed when a hemothorax is suspected.

Flail chest injuries almost invariably require intubation and positive-pressure ventilation. Injuries to the aorta and great vessels or to the trachea and bronchial tree require emergency surgical intervention. See Thoracentesis (p. 12) and Thoracostomy Tube (p. 13) in Chapter 2.

Additional Comments

1. Early notification of surgical trauma team and neurosurgery department is essential.
2. Physical examination points to be stressed include:
   a. Proper evaluation of the pelvis.
   b. Examination of the rectum and genitalia before Foley catheter placement, which is contraindicated in the presence of an overriding prostate, blood at the urethral meatus, or blood in the scrotum.
   c. Examination of the entire patient, including the back.
3. ABG: In a patient with altered mental status and multiple trauma, early assessment for hypoxia and secondary metabolic acidosis.
4. Additional procedures (if indicated; see Chapter 2): Femoral CVL.
5. Call the blood bank early during the resuscitation effort for **whole blood, packed red blood cells**, or **O-negative blood** if necessary (whatever is available immediately).
6. Respiratory compromise resulting from shock or abdominal distention can arise in patients with no pulmonary or cardiac injuries.

REFERENCES

Bender TM et al: Pediatric chest trauma, *J Thorac Imag* 2:60-67, 1987.

Committee on Trauma, American College of Surgeons: *Advanced trauma life support: 1988 reference manual*, Chicago, 1988, American College of Surgeons.

Cooper A, Foltin GL: Thoracic trauma. In Barkin RM: *Pediatric emergency medicine: concepts and clinical practice*, ed 2, St Louis, 1997, Mosby.

Eichelberger MR: Trauma of the airway and thorax, *Pediatr Ann* 16:307-316, 1987.

Templeton JM: Thoracic trauma. In Fleisher GR, Ludwig S, eds: *Textbook of pediatric emergency medicine*, ed 3, Baltimore, 1993, Williams & Wilkins, pp 1143-1166.

29. Multiple Blunt Trauma

CARLOS A. DELGADO

OBJECTIVES

1. Recognize mechanisms for multiple blunt trauma, and be aware that resuscitation begins with the ABCs.
2. Aggressively manage hypovolemic shock with fluid resuscitation.
3. Manage closed head injury.
4. Identify and manage blunt abdominal trauma.
5. Identify and manage blunt thoracic trauma.

Brief Presenting History

An 8-year-old male fell about 20 feet out of his tree house. Approximate 10-minute loss of consciousness at the scene. Brought in by paramedics on a full spine board with the cervical spine immobilized.

Initial Vital Signs

T 37.5° C, P 150, BP 110/70, RR 24.
If asked: Estimated weight 25 kg.

Initial Physical Examination

General appearance: Moaning, intermittently poorly responsive.
If asked: Large contusion and laceration in right parietal region.

- **Airway:** Patent, clear of secretions or evidence of trauma.
- **Breathing:** Symmetric chest excursion, breath sounds full and clear bilaterally.
- **Circulation:** Heart tones normal, capillary refill time 3 seconds, pulses palpable.
- Eyes open to speech, localized response to pain, disoriented and confused (GCS 12).
- Stable midface, no obvious fractures.
- Neck immobilized with a stiff cervical collar.
- Abdomen flat, bowel sounds distant, diffusely tender to palpation. A small ecchymosis is present over the left side of the abdomen.
- Rectum has normal tone, pelvis stable.
- Left upper leg has obvious deformity.

Further History Given on Request

- Previously well child, no hospitalizations.
- No medications, NKDA, tetanus toxoid 2 years previous.

Expected interventions	Complications

1. 100% O$_2$.
2. Monitors (ECG and oximeter).
3. Two large-bore IVs placed.
   Normal saline/Ringer's lactate 20 ml/kg.
4. Laboratory tests: type and cross, CBC,
   amylase, UA.
5. Call for chest, pelvis, C-spine films.
6. Surgery/neurosurgery departments called.
	Vomiting necessitates suction and log roll.
	
	Difficulty starting IV, necessitating IO or CVL
	   placement.

Repeat Vital Signs

P 160, BP 90/40, RR 30, capillary refill time 5 seconds.

Progression

Respirations rapid and shallow. Child is poorly responsive to pain (GCS <7).

Expected interventions	Complications
1. BVM-assisted ventilations. 2. Prepare for rapid sequence intubation. 3. Repeat **normal saline/Ringer's lactate** 20 ml/kg IV. Call for **O-negative blood**.	Vomits if no cricoid pressure. Persistent poor perfusion.

Radiographs

CXR normal, pelvis negative for fracture, C-spine pending.

Progression

Pulses thready, BP 50/P, agonal breathing.
If asked: Abdomen now distended.

Expected interventions	Complications
1. Rapid sequence intubation. Miller no. 2 blade, 6.0 ETT. Preoxygenate with 100% O_2	Right mainstem intubation.
Consider **atropine** 0.02 mg/kg IV. **Lidocaine** 1 mg/kg IV.	
Midazolam 0.1 mg/kg IV.	Tube falls out if not properly taped and cared for.
Vecuronium 0.1 to 0.2 mg/kg IV or **rocuronium** 0.6 to 1 mg/kg IV or **succinylcholine** 1 mg/kg IV after defasciculating **vecuronium** 0.01 mg/kg IV.	
Cricoid pressure.	Vomits if no cricoid pressure or NG tube placed.
Place NG and end-tidal CO_2 monitor. OG if midfacial trauma present. CXR for ETT position.	
2. Hyperventilate (P_{CO_2} 30 to 35).	
3. Begin **whole blood/packed red blood cell** transfusion.	
4. Consider **phenytoin** load 10 to 20 mg/kg IV.	

Additional Potential Complications

1. Asystole caused by hypoperfusion, necessitating chest compressions and pharmacologic resuscitation. Hypovolemia unresponsive to fluid resuscitation caused by ongoing losses from a large hepatic laceration.
2. Seizure caused by increased ICP, intracranial bleeding, or hypoxia, necessitating benzodiazepine control and intubation if not previously performed.
3. C-spine injury or unable to clear C-spine, affecting intubation procedure.
4. Development of hematuria makes renal/GU workup indicated.
5. Increased intracranial pressure requiring head elevation and mannitol. Neurosurgery to place intracranial bolt.
6. Facial trauma and airway obstruction, necessitating needle cricothyrotomy.
7. Unrecognized extremity fracture.

Disposition

If hemodynamically stable, to CT scanner for CT of the head and abdomen. If unstable, immediately to OR for exploratory laparotomy.

Discussion of Objectives

1. *Recognize mechanisms for multiple blunt trauma, and be aware that resuscitation begins with the ABCs.*

Falls are mechanisms associated with major blunt traumatic injuries. Resuscitation begins with the primary survey of the ABCs. Assessment and control of the **airway** with attention to cervical spine immobilization are first. The patient is given 100% oxygen as **breathing** is evaluated. **Circulation** is assessed, two large-bore IVs are placed, and fluid resuscitation is begun. After a rapid neurologic examination the patient is exposed so that all injuries may be evaluated. All problems identified in the primary survey are addressed in the resuscitation phase. In the secondary survey the patient is completely examined and other problems are identified.

During the definitive care phase all injuries are addressed. The trauma surgeons, orthopedic surgeons, and neurosurgeons are responsible for the definitive care phase of trauma. See Cervical Spine Immobilization (p. 11) in Chapter 2 and Trauma (p. 203) in Chapter 4.

2. *Aggressively manage hypovolemic shock with fluid resuscitation.*

Initial fluid resuscitation consists of **isotonic crystalloid** 20 ml/kg given rapidly and repeated if reassessment reveals ongoing losses or hypotension caused by tachycardia and poor perfusion. In pediatric patients low blood pressure is a late finding of shock because of compensatory mechanisms. If patients display tachycardia, diminished pulses, prolonged capillary refill time, or cool mottled skin, hypovolemia must be considered and aggressive fluid resuscitation begun. Persistent hypotension despite **isotonic crystalloid** 40 ml/kg requires the addition of colloid. **Type O-negative whole blood** is used if cross-matched, type-specific whole blood is not available.

Sites of ongoing blood loss must be investigated. The abdomen, retroperitoneum, and pelvis are areas of "silent" bleeding that require evaluation by physical examination and CT scan. Long bone fractures, especially those involving the femurs, can lead to significant bleeding.

Intracranial bleeding typically does not lead to overt hypotension because the cranial vault allows a finite amount of blood loss. However, in infants with open sutures the intracranial space may grow and large amounts of blood may accumulate.

Vasopressors, steroids, and sodium bicarbonate have no role in the initial management of hypovolemic shock in trauma. The "3:1 rule" applies; patients require 300 ml of crystalloid for each 100 ml of blood lost.

3. *Manage closed head injury.*

For GCS of 8 or less (see Appendix F, p. 220).

a. Rapid sequence intubation.

Atropine 0.02 mg/kg IV (used in younger patients to prevent bradycardia induced by vagal stimulation).

Lidocaine 1 mg/kg IV.

Midazolam 0.1 to 0.3 mg/kg IV.

Thiopental may exacerbate hypotension and should not be used in this case.

Vecuronium 0.1 to 0.2 mg/kg IV or **rocuronium** 0.6 to 1 mg/kg IV.

Succinylcholine may result in ICP elevation but is not absolutely contraindicated in head injuries. A defasciculating dose of **vecuronium** 0.01 mg/kg IV is given before succinylcholine. Succinylcholine is contraindicated in crush injuries, severe burns (hyperkalemia), glaucoma (increased ocular pressure), penetrating eye injuries, and significant neuromuscular disease. (See Rapid Sequence Intubation [p. 10] in Chapter 2.)

  b. Hyperventilation. Patients are hyperventilated to decrease intracranial pressure, with a P_{CO_2} goal of approximately 30 to 35.

  c. Mannitol as an osmotic diuretic (use is contraindicated in hypotension). In the management of a patient with increased intracranial pressure the goal is to maintain cerebral perfusion pressure (CPP):

$$CPP = MAP - ICP \ (MAP = \text{mean arterial pressure}; ICP = \text{intracranial pressure})$$

Thus volume resuscitation, maintenance of mean arterial pressure, is vital. (See Increased Intracranial Pressure [p. 196] in Chapter 4 and mock code 26, Closed Head Injury [p. 129].)

4. *Identify and manage blunt abdominal trauma.*

The management of BAT begins with attention to the ABCs, emphasizing aggressive volume resuscitation as discussed previously. Evaluation of the hematocrit offers information about amount of bleeding but may not show a significant decline initially. Urinalysis is performed to investigate possible renal trauma. Blood in the urine is also a nonspecific marker for significant abdominal trauma that does not necessarily involve the kidneys. An elevated amylase level is indicative of pancreatic trauma, but the concentration may be high with injuries to salivary glands and also may not be elevated initially. The CT scan of the abdomen remains the gold standard for investigating BAT in pediatric patients. Limitations include evaluation of the duodenum for hematoma and emergency operative evaluation of a hemodynamically unstable patient.

Diagnostic peritoneal lavage (DPL) is used in adult BAT to evaluate the peritoneal cavity for bleeding. Indications for DPL in the pediatric population are limited because most causes of pediatric intraperitoneal bleeding, such as liver and splenic lacerations, are now managed nonoperatively. One potential indication is the hypotensive pediatric patient with head and abdominal injuries. A positive DPL necessitates immediate exploratory laparotomy. If the DPL is negative, the patient may be sent to the CT scanner for evaluation of the head with further volume resuscitation.

Studies are under way to evaluate emergency diagnostic abdominal ultrasound as a means of ascertaining whether significant intraabdominal fluid (blood) is present. Use of emergency abdominal ultrasound in adult centers is becoming widespread, but it is not yet used routinely in children.

The cornerstone of management of BAT is adequate volume resuscitation, as discussed previously, and aggressive diagnostic evaluation of the causes of shock. Much of pediatric BAT is managed nonoperatively, but in patients with ongoing blood loss surgical intervention may be lifesaving. (See mock code 27, Blunt Abdominal Trauma [p. 135].)

5. *Identify and manage blunt thoracic trauma.*

The presence of unilateral decreased breath sounds suggests pneumothorax, hemothorax, or hemopneumothorax. When desaturation occurs despite maximal oxygen delivery, or hypotension despite aggressive fluid resuscitation, surgical or needle aspiration of the chest is indicated. In this case there is no time for confirmation of diagnosis by chest radiograph. Deviation of the trachea or cardiac sounds should be sought as evidence of a tension pneumothorax. Needle thoracentesis should be performed by means of a large-bore IV catheter connected to a three-way stopcock and 60 ml syringe. The needle should be inserted into the thoracic cavity over the second rib in the midclavicular line.

After palliation by needle thoracentesis a chest tube is placed over the fourth rib in the midaxillary line. If no improvement is seen, the tube is redirected posteriorly in an attempt to remove blood. Needling the chest may not be sufficient to extract blood; a chest tube should be placed when a hemothorax is suspected.

Flail chest injuries almost invariably require intubation and positive-pressure ventilation. Injuries to the aorta and great vessels or to the trachea and bronchial tree require emergency surgical intervention. See Thoracentesis (p. 12) and Thoracostomy Tube (p. 13) in Chapter 2 and mock code 28, Blunt Thoracic Trauma (p. 140).

Additional Comments

1. Early notification of surgical trauma team and neurosurgery is essential.
2. Physical examination points to be stressed include:
   a. Proper evaluation of the pelvis.
   b. Rectal and genitalia examination before Foley catheter placement, which is contraindicated in the presence of an overriding prostate, blood at the urethral meatus, or blood in the scrotum.
   c. Examination of entire patient, including the back.
3. ABG: In a patient with altered mental status and multiple trauma, early assessment for hypoxia and secondary metabolic acidosis.
4. Procedures (if indicated; see Chapter 2).
   a. Femoral CVL.
   b. Chest thoracostomy tube.
5. Call the blood bank for whole blood, packed red blood cells, or O-negative blood (whatever is available immediately) early during the resuscitation effort if necessary.
6. Respiratory compromise can arise in patients with no pulmonary or cardiac injuries resulting from shock or abdominal distention.

REFERENCES

Committee on Trauma, American College of Surgeons: *Advanced trauma life support*, ed 5, Chicago, 1993.

Fitzmaurice LS: Approach to multiple trauma. In Barkin RM: *Pediatric emergency medicine, concepts and clinical practice*, ed 2, St Louis, 1997, Mosby.

Kaufman BA, Dacey RG: Acute management of closed head injury in childhood, *Pediatr Ann* 23:18-28, 1994.

Manary MJ, Jaffe DM: Cervical spine injuries in children, *Pediatr Ann* 25:423-428, 1996.

Nordenholz KE et al: Ultrasound in the evaluation and management of blunt abdominal trauma, *Ann Emerg Med* 29:357-366, 1997.

Saladino RA, Lund DP: Abdominal trauma. In Fleisher GR, Ludwig S, eds: *Textbook of pediatric emergency medicine*, ed 3, Baltimore, 1993, Williams & Wilkins, pp 1167-1174.

Templeton JM: Thoracic trauma. In Fleisher GR, Ludwig S, eds: *Textbook of pediatric emergency medicine*, ed 3, Baltimore, 1993, Williams & Wilkins, pp 1143-1166.

Ziegler MM, Templeton JM: Major trauma. In Fleisher GR, Ludwig S, eds: *Textbook of pediatric emergency medicine*, ed 3, Baltimore, 1993, Williams & Wilkins, pp 1089-1102.

30. Penetrating Trauma

ALLAN DOCTOR

OBJECTIVES

1. Manage the airway in penetrating and blunt neck trauma.
2. Aggressively manage penetrating chest trauma.
3. Manage hypovolemic shock.

Brief Presenting History

July 4th. A 10-year-old boy playing with fireworks accidentally creates an explosion near an old picket fence, which shatters. The child is struck by several large wooden fragments, which are stabilized in place by Emergency Medical Services en route.

Initial Vital Signs

P 138, BP 70/P, RR 54 (labored).
If asked: T 37.3° C (T), estimated weight 30 kg.

Initial Physical Examination

General appearance: Frightened, pale child in marked respiratory distress.
If asked:
- **Airway:** Clear, no facial or oral trauma, saliva bloody, and voice hoarse. Six-inch wooden splinter entering neck anterior to left sternocleidomastoid muscle just under angle of mandible, ecchymosis and abrasion over anterior neck (larynx), subcutaneous emphysema present, neck veins distended.
- **Breathing:** Absence of breath sounds on the right. Similar-sized splinter entering the right chest just lateral and inferior to nipple.
- **Circulation:** Radial pulse thready, capillary refill time 3 to 4 seconds.
- Alert, panicky, but GCS 15.
- Abdomen firm, but patient screaming continuously. No external sign of abdominal, perineal, extremity, or back trauma.

Further History Given on Request

Previously well child, no medications, NKDA.
- Last tetanus toxoid at 4 years of age.

Expected interventions	*Complications*

1. 100% O_2, suction airway.
    Immobilize neck without dislodging projectiles.
2. Place monitors (ECG, pulse oximeter).
3. Needle thoracentesis, right side of chest.
    Prepare for chest tube placement.
4. Two large-bore IVs.
    Normal saline 20 ml/kg rapid IV bolus.
    Laboratory tests: Type and cross, Hct.
5. Call for **O-negative blood**.
6. Call for CXR, lateral neck film.
7. Contact trauma surgeons.
See Thoracentesis (p. 12) and Thoracostomy Tube (p. 13) in Chapter 2.
	Respiratory arrest if thoracentesis not performed immediately.
	Reaccumulation of tension pneumothorax, requires repeat needle thoracentesis and chest tube placement.

Progression

Needle thoracostomy results in a large rush of air and improved right-sided breath sounds.

Repeat Vital Signs

P 110, BP 95/55, RR 45, capillary refill time 3 to 4 seconds.

Expected interventions	*Complications*

1. Repeat **normal saline** 20 ml/kg IV.
 	
2. Place right-sided 32 Fr chest tube.
    Fentanyl 2 μg/kg IV.
    Midazolam 0.1 mg/kg IV.
	Failure to place chest tube results in hypotension and respiratory failure.

Radiographs

Lateral neck: Soft tissue emphysema caused by penetrating pharyngeal injury.
CXR: Right chest tube in good position, no extraparenchymal air.

Progression	Expected interventions
Option 1	
Perfusion improves with volume resuscitation, but stridor and increased RR develop. Chest tube produces 10 ml serosanguineous fluid. P 110, BP 95/55, RR 55, Hct 40.	1. Awake intubation. Suction secretions. Miller or Mac no. 2, 6.0 or 6.5 ETT. **Midazolam** 0.1 mg/kg IV. Cricoid pressure. 2. Place NG tube and end-tidal CO_2 monitor. 3. CXR for ETT position.
Option 2	
Patient develops stridor, bloody secretions in mouth, becomes responsive to painful stimuli only. Capillary refill time 4 seconds. Chest tube produces 500 ml of blood. P 150, BP 65/P, RR 60, Hct 30.	1. Awake intubation. Suction secretions. Miller or Mac no. 2, 6.0 or 6.5 ETT. **Midazolam** 0.1 mg/kg IV. Cricoid pressure. 2. Place NG tube and end-tidal CO_2 monitor. 3. CXR for ETT position. 4. Transfuse **PRBCs** 20 ml/kg IV, **O-negative blood** if not cross-matched.

Progression	Expected interventions
Option 1	
Patient's condition stabilizes with intubation.	1. Tetanus toxoid. 2. Antibiotics.
Option 2	
Patient's condition stabilizes with blood transfusion and intubation, *or* Intubation is unsuccessful.	1. Tetanus toxoid. 2. Antibiotics. 3. Percutaneous cricothyrotomy. 4. OR for surgical airway.

Additional Potential Complications

1. If a barbiturate is used for sedation, the patient becomes acutely more hypotensive, leading to cardiac arrest.
2. Persistent hypotension results from penetrating hepatic trauma. This emphasizes the point that all penetrating chest trauma below the nipple line has the potential to become penetrating abdominal trauma because of diaphragmatic excursion.

3. The patient becomes combative during painful procedures (e.g., chest tube placement) if no analgesics or sedation is used.

Disposition

OR for exploration of the neck and removal of the splinter in the right side of the chest.

Discussion of Objectives

1. *Manage the airway in penetrating and blunt neck trauma.*

   Perform the primary survey, recognizing pharyngeal hemorrhage that requires suctioning and injuries to the neck that may lead to acute airway obstruction.

   Penetrating neck trauma may lead to hypopharyngeal bleeding and airway obstruction. Projectiles found in the neck should not be removed, since this may lead to increased bleeding from vessels that have tamponaded. Immobilization of the cervical spine is performed in a manner to accommodate protruding projectiles. The mouth and pharynx are suctioned, and the airway is assessed. Blunt laryngeal injury may result in airway obstruction caused by laryngeal injury (fracture or edema of the larynx or hematoma at or below the level of vocal cords) or a pharyngeal mass (hematoma). The examiner should look for outward signs such as contusions or subcutaneous emphysema over the anterior neck, as well as stridor and hoarseness.

   When a difficult intubation is anticipated because of laryngeal trauma, awake laryngoscopy should be attempted, followed either by awake intubation if the view is difficult or by rapid sequence intubation if access to the airway appears relatively unobstructed.

   Note: Anytime a difficult intubation is anticipated, it is prudent to notify appropriate airway management services (anesthesia, ENT) immediately. Fiberoptics may be helpful in these types of intubations, and the need for emergency cricothyrotomy must be anticipated.

2. *Aggressively manage penetrating chest trauma.*

   As in the neck, projectiles found in the chest or abdomen should not be removed during initial resuscitation. In a patient who has penetrating chest trauma, shock, and unilateral absence of breath sounds with distended neck veins, four possible etiologies must be considered:

   a. Tension pneumothorax.

   b. Massive hemothorax.

   c. Simple pneumothorax plus extrathoracic hemorrhage.

   d. Simple pneumothorax and cardiac tamponade.

   With this presentation, needle thoracostomy followed by chest tube placement should be undertaken immediately. Aggressive fluid resuscitation should also be initiated. Aggressive evaluation must be undertaken to identify sites of blood loss discrete from the chest.

   All the preceding conditions eventually will require tube thoracostomy, but it should be emphasized that minimal additional risk is incurred by performing needle thoracostomy, which may be lifesaving (especially in cases of tension pneumothorax).

   Chest tubes must never be placed through openings in the thorax caused by penetrating trauma.

3. *Manage hypovolemic shock.*

   Aggressive volume resuscitation is essential for hypotension in any type of traumatic injury. In patients with penetrating trauma, large volumes of blood may be lost rapidly and volume resuscitation with isotonic crystalloid should be initiated immediately, followed by the administration of colloid.

After evacuation of a tension pneumothorax the persistence of hypovolemic shock indicates ongoing hemorrhage in the chest that is not being evacuated or bleeding at a distal site. Cardiac tamponade must also be considered.

Aggressive volume resuscitation is the first step in the management of both conditions. If penetrating trauma (except gunshot wounds) is lateral to the nipple, cardiac injury is rare and hemorrhage (especially occult abdominal injury, in the absence of a hemothorax) should be suspected as the cause.

Suspected tamponade in a victim of penetrating thoracic trauma is beyond the scope of this scenario and should be managed with extremely aggressive volume resuscitation, including the administration of **O-negative blood**, until the arrival of a surgeon.

Universal donor blood (O-negative) should be used immediately in crisis situations when there is no time for cross-matching. Because the A, B, and Rh antigens are absent, theoretically this blood can be administered to nearly any recipient.

Some donors with **O-negative blood** have high titers of anti-A or anti-B antibodies in their serum. In military experience with whole blood transfusion, blood from these donors has caused hemolytic transfusion reactions. This complication is not a concern with the use of packed red cell transfusions. If 5 to 10 minutes is available, type-specific blood should be used instead.

Additional Comments

1. Repetition of the primary survey after each intervention is essential for recognizing and managing the complications of penetrating chest and neck trauma, as well as blunt laryngeal injury.
   a. Expanding pharyngeal hematoma.
   b. Hypopharyngeal bleeding.
   c. Tension pneumothorax.
   d. Massive hemothorax.
   e. Concealed intraabdominal hemorrhage.
2. Antibiotic coverage for penetrating neck injuries must be broad spectrum in nature to cover *Staphylococcus, Streptococcus*, and anaerobes.

REFERENCES

American College of Surgeons, Committee on Trauma: *Advanced trauma life support: program for physicians*, Chicago, 1993, American College of Surgeons.

Dailey RH, Simon B, Young GP, Stewart RD: *The airway: emergency management*, St Louis, 1992, Mosby.

Fuhrman GM, Steig FH, Buerk CA: Blunt laryngeal trauma: classification and management, *J Trauma* 30:87-92, 1990.

Lefebre J: Seven years experience with group O unmatched red blood cells in a regional trauma unit, *Ann Emerg Med* 16:1344-1351, 1987.

Myer CM, Orobello P, Cotton RT, Bratcher GO: Blunt laryngeal trauma in children, *Laryngoscope* 97:1043-1048, 1987.

Saletta JD et al: Penetrating trauma of the neck, *J Trauma* 16:579-597, 1976.

ENVIRONMENTAL EMERGENCIES
31. Burns and Smoke Inhalation

MARK G. ROBACK

OBJECTIVES

1. Recognize and manage the airway altered by heat and smoke inhalation.
2. Recognize and manage the complications of severe burns and smoke inhalation.
3. Recognize and manage underlying trauma-related injuries.

Brief Presenting History

An 8-year-old male was found on the ground beneath a second-story window of a burning house.

Initial Vital Signs

P 150, RR 32, BP 100/60.
If asked: T 36.5° C (R), pulse oximetry 95%, estimated weight 25 kg.

Initial Physical Examination

General appearance: Red-faced child thrashing on a hard board.
If asked: Clothes blackened and charred.
- **Airway:** Patent but carbonaceous material in mouth and nose.
- **Breathing:** Fast and shallow, breaths sounds equal with occasional expiratory wheeze and crackles.
- **Circulation:** Tachycardic, capillary refill time 3 seconds centrally, pulses 1+/2+ radial and femoral.
- Opens eyes to speech (3), responds inappropriately (3), nonspecific withdrawal from pain (4), Glasgow Coma Scale score = 10.
- Head, hair burned, boggy to palpation over right occipital region, eyebrows singed.
- Erythema with blisters over neck and arms; skin over the chest extending to the back is pale and leathery.
- Pupils 4 mm, reactive to 2 mm bilaterally.
- Abdomen nondistended, occasional bowel sounds, soft.
- Pelvis intact, rectal with normal tone, stool heme negative.
- Back has erythematous skin, becoming white laterally.
- No obvious extremity abnormalities, but hands and feet becoming edematous.

Further History Given on Request

- History of RAD, taking albuterol inhaler PRN.
- No other medications. Last tetanus toxoid at 18 months of age.

Expected interventions	Complications
1. 100% O_2 by nonrebreather.	
2. Cervical spine immobilization with hard board.	Vomiting, requires log roll and suction.
3. ECG monitor and pulse oximetry.	
4. IV access, two large-bore catheters.	IV access through burned skin if necessary.
Ringer's lactate or **normal saline** 20 ml/kg IV.	
5. Rapid sequence intubation.	
6.0 ETT, no. 2 or 3 Miller/Mac.	Failure to control airway leads to progressive respiratory distress, stridor, and respiratory arrest.
Consider **atropine** 0.02 mg/kg IV.	
Midazolam 0.1 mg/kg IV.	
Fentanyl 2 to 5 µg/kg IV.	
Vecuronium 0.1 to 0.2 mg/kg IV or **rocuronium** 0.6 to 1 mg/kg IV.	Supraglottic edema present, necessitating smaller (5.5) ETT.
Cricoid pressure.	Vomiting if no cricoid pressure.
Lidocaine 1 mg/kg IV if head injury suspected.	
Place NG and end-tidal CO_2 monitor.	If endotracheal intubation unsuccessful, percutaneous cricothyrotomy required.
6. Laboratory tests: ABG, CBC, electrolytes, carboxyhemoglobin and cyanide levels, type and screen.	
7. CXR, lateral neck, and pelvis films ordered.	
8. Foley catheter placed, UA requested.	Delay in airway control leads to progressive airway edema and obstruction.
9. **Tetanus** toxoid 0.5 ml IM.	
10. Alert trauma team, surgery department.	

Repeat Vital Signs

HR 120, BP 95/50.

Laboratory Findings

ABG pH 7.22, P_{CO_2} 60, P_{O_2} 56, Na 139, K 4.2, HCO_3 17, glucose 159, Hct 37.

Progression

Patient becoming progressively more difficult to bag. Poor chest excursion, bilateral decreased breath sounds.

Expected interventions	Complications
1. Escharotomy, chest.	Failure to recognize need for escharotomy leads to respiratory arrest.

◆

Progression

Significant generalized edema develops, making the patient progressively more difficult to bag. Oxygen saturations drop to the high 80s. Capillary refill time is 3 to 4 seconds. HR 135, BP 90/45.

Expected interventions	Complications

1. Add positive end-expiratory pressure (PEEP).
2. Seek additional IV access, CVL.
3. Repeat **RL** or **NS** 20 ml/kg IV.
 	
   Consider **5% albumin** 20 ml/kg IV.
   Consider **dopamine** 2 to 10 μg/kg/min.
4. Recheck electrolytes.
	Overaggressive bagging leads to a pneumothorax.
	
	Failure to fluid resuscitate adequately leads to cardiovascular collapse.

◆

Progression

Secondary survey reveals a 6 cm depressed, boggy area on the right side of the occiput. Abdomen becomes tense. Capillary refill time remains 3 to 4 seconds. BP 85/40 despite aggressive fluid resuscitation.

Expected interventions	Complications

1. Raise the head of the bed.
2. **Lorazepam** 0.05 to 0.1 mg/kg IV.
   Load with **phenytoin** 10 to 20 mg/kg IV.
3. Hyperventilate to P_{CO_2} level of 30 to 35.
4. Continue aggressive volume replacement.
 	
   5% albumin 20 ml/kg IV.
   Consider **O-negative blood**.
	Generalized tonic-clonic seizure.
	
	Failure to fluid resuscitate adequately leads to cardiovascular collapse.

◆

Options

1. Abdominal distention and poor response to volume replacement strongly suggest intraabdominal bleeding. If the patient is hemodynamically stable, send to radiology department for CT of abdomen and head. If the patient is unstable, move directly to OR.

Additional Potential Complications

1. Failure to paralyze, sedate, and provide pain medication properly leads to the patient's awakening and extubating self. Reintubation attempts fail because of airway edema, necessitating cricothyrotomy.
2. Failure to treat shock aggressively with volume replacement leads to cardiovascular collapse and arrest.

Disposition

If the patient becomes hemodynamically stable, to radiology department for CT of the head and abdomen. If the patient is hemodynamically unstable, to OR for exploratory laparotomy.

Discussion of Objectives

1. *Recognize and manage the airway altered by heat and smoke inhalation.*
   Inhalation of hot gas results in burns of the pharynx and upper airway. Edema may progress over the next several hours. To prevent significant morbidity and mortality caused by airway obstruction, the team must control the airway early in the course. Evidence of airway burns, including facial or intraoral erythema, singed nose or facial hairs, or carbonaceous debris, is an indication for aggressive control of the airway via endotracheal intubation. Failure to secure the airway may lead to airway obstruction, necessitating cricothyrotomy. (See Airway [p. 9] in Chapter 2.)
2. *Recognize and manage the complications of severe burns and smoke inhalation.*
   Hypoxia is the most common cause of death in the first hour after the burn. Carbon monoxide (CO) poisoning from smoke inhalation resulting in insufficient oxygen delivery is common. Maintenance of adequate oxygenation and ventilation is essential. Careful attention must be paid to the patient's level of consciousness. Continuous pulse oximetry and frequent arterial blood gas determinations are also helpful in monitoring the level of hypoxia, hypercarbia, and CO poisoning. *Note:* Pulse oximetry readings may be falsely normal in CO poisoning.
   The fluid and electrolyte balance may be severely altered in patients with significant burns. Initial aggressive fluid resuscitation using isotonic crystalloid solution such as **Ringer's lactate** or **normal saline** is advised. Urine output should be maintained at 1 ml/kg/hr minimum. Electrolyte levels should be measured frequently because ongoing losses could be great.
   Capillary leak in a severely burned patient leads to anasarca and pulmonary edema. At least two sites of IV access should be secured early in the course before edema makes this task more difficult. Vasopressors may be necessary to reduce shock from this mechanism after volume resuscitation. Volume resuscitation is vital when occult traumatic bleeding is suspected. Positive end-expiratory pressure (PEEP) improves oxygenation in patients with pulmonary edema, but barotrauma is a complication to be considered.
   Eschar formation, especially in circumferential distributions, may lead to compromised blood flow to digits or extremities. With full-thickness burns and eschar formation around the thorax, severe respiratory compromise may occur. In this instance, escharotomy may be lifesaving.
3. *Recognize and manage underlying trauma-related injuries.*
   Traumatic injuries resulting from falls and from falling debris must always be suspected in fires. Management begins with immobilization of the cervical spine. Careful examination of the head,

chest, abdomen, pelvis, back, and extremities for evidence of trauma is essential. Aggressive fluid resuscitation is often required, followed by diagnostic CT and surgical intervention as indicated. See Trauma (p. 203) in Chapter 4.

Additional Comments

1. For management of closed head injuries and multiple blunt trauma see mock codes 26 (p. 129) and 29 (p. 146).

REFERENCES

Coren C: Burn injuries in children, *Pediatr Ann* 16:328-339, 1987.
Finkelstein JL et al: Pediatric burns: an overview, *Pediatr Clin North Am* 39:1145-1163, 1992.
Parish RA: Smoke inhalation and carbon monoxide poisoning in children, *Pediatr Emerg Care* 2:36-41, 1986.
Schiller WR: Burn management in children, *Pediatr Ann* 25:431-438, 1996.

32. Drowning—Hypothermia

RICHARD SALADINO

OBJECTIVES

1. Recognize the priorities of the management of drowning.
2. Recognize and treat hypothermia and complications of hypothermia.
3. Consider potential associated problems: intoxication, head injury, cervical spine injury.

Brief Presenting History

An 8-year-old boy falls through the ice while skating. He is rescued by bystanders after 10 minutes in the water. CPR is begun at the scene; EMTs arrive after 20 minutes. Full arrest at the scene.

Initial Vital Signs

HR 0, RR 0: bag-mask ventilation.
If asked: T 31.3° C, estimated weight 25 kg.

Initial Physical Examination

General appearance: Palc, lips white, appears dead.
If asked:
- **Airway:** Airway patent, trachea midline.
- **Breathing:** Breath sounds full and equal with bagging.
- **Circulation:** Pulseless, capillary refill time 5 seconds, skin very cold.
- Pupils dilated, fixed.
- Abdomen distended.

Further History Given on Request

Previously well, no medications, NKDA.

Expected interventions	Complications
1. Begin CPR. BVM with 100% O_2. Chest compression attempts not effective. C-spine immobilization.	If no warming, patient progresses to V-tach without a pulse, necessitating defibrillation.
2. ECG monitor, oximeter.	IV attempts unsuccessful, necessitating IO placement.
3. Endotracheal intubation. 6.0 cuffed ETT. NG tube and end-tidal CO_2 monitor. CXR for ETT placement.	Right mainstem intubation.
4. Large-bore IV catheters. Rapid glucose, ABG, Hct. **Normal saline/Ringer's lactate** 20 ml/kg IV/IO.	ETT falls out if not properly handled.
5. Begin warming. Warm inspired oxygen. Warm IVF, with short tubing. Thermal blanket/warming lights. Warm **NS** lavage per NG/bladder irrigation (see Additional Comments no. 3). Chest tube/thoracotomy warm lavage.	Vomiting if no cricoid pressure or NG.
7. **Epinephrine** 0.1 ml/kg, 1:10,000 IV/IO or 1:1000 ETT.	
8. Call for trauma team/surgical consult.	

Laboratory Results

Hct 36, ABG: pH 7.02, P_{CO_2} 60, P_{O_2} 180, base excess -12.

Repeat Vital Signs

T 34.4° C, HR 50, BP 75/40, pulse oximetry 88%.

Progression

V-tach with rewarming, decreased lung compliance, increased difficulty bagging.

Expected interventions	Complications
1. Continue CPR until warm (>32° C) or HR >100.	Ventricular tachycardia.
2. **Epinephrine** 1:10,000, 0.1 ml/kg.	
3. Cardiovert 1 J/kg, synchronized if pulse present. **Lidocaine** 1 mg/kg bolus, drip 20 to 50 µg/kg/min.	Persistent V-tach, loss of pulses.
4. Defibrillate 2 J/kg, asynchronized mode.	
5. Treat hypotension. Repeat 20 ml/kg **Ringer's lactate** bolus. **Dopamine** 10 µg/kg/min.	Decreasing oxygenation.
6. Increase PEEP ≥4 cm H₂O.	Pneumothorax, acute hypotension.
7. Listen to chest for breath sounds. Needle the side without breath sounds (see Thoracentesis in Chapter 2). Place chest tube.	

Additional Potential Complications

1. Persistent ventricular tachycardia or decompensation to ventricular fibrillation if cardioversion or defibrillation attempted when the temperature is less than 32° C.
2. Persistent hypotension if fluid resuscitation is inadequate.
3. Seizure caused by undetected head trauma or hypoxia.

Disposition

ICU when warmed, rhythm stable.

Discussion of Objectives

1. *Recognize the priorities of the management of drowning.*

   The ABCs of resuscitation, including immobilization of the cervical spine, must be addressed first. Approximately 90% of drowning victims aspirate fluid. All patients have hypoxemia. Hypothermia must be suspected and addressed in all patients, even victims of warm water drownings (see no. 2 below).

   There are differences between saltwater and fresh water drownings. Aspiration of large volumes of saltwater leads acutely to relative hypovolemia with concentration of extracellular electrolytes. Conversely, fresh water aspiration results in acute hypervolemia with dilution of extracellular electrolytes. In cases of fresh water aspiration, with rapid redistribution of fluid and the development of pulmonary edema, hypovolemic shock develops rapidly. Both fresh water and saltwater aspiration victims require aggressive fluid resuscitation.

   Endotracheal intubation with consideration of positive end-expiratory pressure (PEEP) for treatment of pulmonary edema is the single most effective treatment in reversing hypoxemia, regardless of water type. With fluid resuscitation and underlying pulmonary insult, pulmonary edema and hypoxia can be expected to develop.

2. *Recognize and treat hypothermia and complications of hypothermia.*

Core rewarming: Methods typically used include warmed oxygen, thermal blanket, warming lights, warmed IV fluids (the shortest possible length of IV tubing should be used to ensure the efficacy of this method), gastric and bladder lavage with warm fluids, and chest tube and thoracotomy lavage with warm sterile saline. Cardiopulmonary bypass is the most aggressive method of rewarming.

Recognize and treat ventricular tachycardia and ventricular fibrillation. Cardioactive medications and cardioversion or defibrillation attempts typically are ineffective when the core temperature is ≤32° C. Patients should be warmed, administered epinephrine, and then shocked. *Note:* Standard thermometers read only down to 34° C. The mock code may be made more rigorous by giving the temperature as 34° C and forcing the team to realize that this reading is not accurate.

In some cases rapid, severe hypothermia may have protective effects on the brain by decreasing metabolic needs. For this reason resuscitative efforts should never be terminated until the victim has been warmed. Traditionally, "You are not dead until you are warm and dead."

3. *Consider potential associated problems: intoxication, head injury, cervical spine injury.*

Consider and treat intoxications with alcohol and other drugs.

Consider and treat traumatic injuries that may not be readily recognizable because of hypothermia and altered mental status. (See Trauma [p. 203] in Chapter 4.)

Consider underlying medical conditions that may play a role: seizures or cardiac disorders.

Additional Comments

1. Goals:
   a. Establish an airway for positive-pressure ventilation and oxygenation.
   b. Perform core rewarming (essential during CPR).
2. Early notification of the trauma team and ICU staff is essential, especially if hypothermia is refractory to aggressive rewarming and necessitates lavage by chest tube or thoracotomy or cardiopulmonary bypass.
3. GI warming by nasogastric tube lavage is controversial. It has been argued that direct stimulation of irritable myocardium may lead to ventricular fibrillation.

REFERENCES

Brunette DD et al: Comparison of gastric lavage and thoracic cavity lavage in the treatment of severe hypothermia in dogs, *Ann Emerg Med* 16:1222-1227, 1987.

Corneli HM: Accidental hypothermia, *J Pediatr* 120:671-679, 1992.

Gonzalez-Rothi RJ: Near drowning: consensus and controversies in pulmonary and cerebral resuscitation, *Heart Lung* 16:474-482, 1987.

Hall KN, Syverud SA: Closed thoracic cavity lavage in the treatment of severe hypothermia in human beings, *Ann Emerg Med* 19:204-206, 1990.

Modell JH: Drowning, *N Engl J Med* 328:253-256, 1993.

O'Conner D: Use of peritoneal dialysis in severely hypothermic patients, *Ann Emerg Med* 15:104-105, 1986.

Orlowski JP, Abulleil MM, Phillips JM: The hemodynamic and cardiovascular effects of near-drowning in hypotonic, isotonic, or hypertonic solutions, *Ann Emerg Med* 18:1044-1049, 1989.

33. Heat Stroke
HOLLY PERRY

OBJECTIVES
1. Recognize the presentation of heat stroke.
2. Manage heat stroke.
3. Manage the complications of heat stroke.

Brief Presenting History

A 1-year-old male has been brought in by his 16-year-old baby-sitter because he was "acting funny."

Initial Vital Signs

HR 200, RR 60, BP 80/P.
If asked: T 42.6° C (R), estimated weight 10 kg.

Initial Physical Examination

General appearance: Lethargic, unresponsive child with diffusely flushed, erythematous, dry skin.
If asked:
- **Airway:** Patent.
- **Breathing:** Breathing unlabored but shallow, breath sounds clear.
- **Circulation:** Tachycardic but no murmurs, capillary refill time 4 to 5 seconds, pulses full and equal.
- Head normocephalic and atraumatic, pupils equal, reactive 3 to 2 mm.
- Abdomen has normal active bowel sounds, soft, no masses.
- Skin flushed but no discrete rash.
- Neurologic: Unresponsive to pain but nonfocal.

Further History Given on Request

Child has had some vomiting and diarrhea for the past 2 days. The baby-sitter drove to the grocery store and left the baby in his carseat for "just a minute" while she ran in for a soda pop with the car locked and the windows rolled up. The weather is sunny, temperature 95° F.

Expected interventions	Complications
1. 100% oxygen.	
2. Monitors (ECG, pulse oximeter, rectal temperature probe).	Vomits.
3. Remove patient's clothes. Institute cooling measures—ice, wet sheet with fan.	
4. Two large-bore IVs. **Normal saline** 20 ml/kg IV/IO.	Unable to obtain IV access, necessitating IO.
5. Laboratory tests: Rapid glucose, ABG, CBC, electrolytes, blood culture, coagulation, UA/UC.	
6. Empiric antibiotic: **Ceftriaxone** 100 mg/kg IV/IO.	

Repeat Vital Signs

T 42.5° C, RR 66, pulse oximetry 87%.

Laboratory Results

Rapid glucose 126, ABG: pH 7.22, P_{CO_2} 25, P_{O_2} 65.

Progression

Capillary refill time 4 seconds, agonal respirations develop.

Expected interventions	Complications
1. Assist BVM. Cricoid pressure.	Vomits if no cricoid pressure.
2. Prepare for rapid sequence intubation.	
3. Continue aggressive cooling measures.	IO infiltrates.
4. Place second IO, attempt CVL. Repeat **normal saline** 20 ml/kg IV/IO bolus.	

Progression

Patient begins having a generalized tonic-clonic seizure.

Expected interventions	Complications
1. **Lorazepam** 0.05 to 0.1 mg/kg IV/IO.	Seizure stops briefly, then resumes.
2. Repeat **lorazepam** 0.05 to 0.1 mg/kg IV/IO.	
3. **Phenytoin** load 15 to 20 mg/kg over 20 minutes.	Cardiovascular collapse if dilantin given rapidly.
4. Continue aggressive cooling.	

Progression

Seizure stops, patient is apneic.

Expected interventions	Complications
1. Rapid sequence intubation.	
4.0 ETT, Miller no. 1 blade.	Right mainstem intubation.
Atropine 0.2 mg IV/IO.	Tube falls out if not properly taped and cared for.
+/−**Vecuronium** 0.1 to 0.2 mg/kg IV/IO.	
Cricoid pressure.	Vomits if no cricoid pressure.
3. Place NG and end-tidal CO_2 monitor.	No NG leads to abdominal distention and
4. CXR for ETT position.	desaturation.
6. Place Foley catheter.	

Repeat Vital Signs

Pulse oximetry after intubation 95%, BP 60/P, T 42° C.

Progression

Capillary refill time 4 seconds.

Expected Interventions

1. **Dobutamine** 5 to 10 µg/kg/min IV continuous infusion.
2. Continue aggressive cooling.

Progression

Blood pressure and perfusion improve, patient cooling down.

Additional Potential Complications

1. Disseminated intravascular coagulation develops, necessitating administration of fresh frozen plasma.
2. Myoglobinuria is managed by an isotonic fluid bolus to maintain urine output of 1 to 2 ml/kg/hr. Insertion of a Foley catheter is recommended.

Disposition

ICU.

Discussion of Objectives

1. *Recognize the presentation of heat stroke.*

   Heat illness is a spectrum of disease ranging from muscular cramps to heat stroke. Heat stroke is a life-threatening emergency characterized by hyperpyrexia (temperature >41° C), dry, hot, flushed skin, and neurologic abnormalities, including confusion, obtundation, focal deficits, and seizures. Additional physical findings are tachycardia, tachypnea, and potentially hypotension.

   In addition to heat stroke the differential diagnosis of hyperpyrexia and neurologic abnormalities includes central nervous system infections, endocrinologic emergencies such as "thyroid storm," and drug reactions or ingestions (sympathomimetics, anticholinergics, antidopaminergics, salicylates, and drugs of abuse). Neuroleptic malignant syndrome and malignant hyperthermia that occur in genetically susceptible people exposed to certain drugs are different because there is intense muscular rigidity in addition to hyperpyrexia.

2. *Manage heat stroke.*

   Treatment begins with attention to the ABCs and then focuses on rapid cooling. After removal of all clothing, cooling should be instituted immediately if heat stroke is suspected. Cooling may be lifesaving and is not harmful if the hyperpyrexia has a cause different from heat stroke. The goal is to bring the temperature to 39.5° C within 1 hour.

   The core temperature should be monitored continuously with either a rectal or an esophageal probe so that cooling is not excessive. The best cooling method remains controversial. Ice packs on the groin, axillae, and neck alone are seldom adequate. Packing the entire patient in ice leads to more rapid cooling but makes the condition of the patient difficult to assess and may lead to shivering, which results in further generation of heat.

   Shivering may be controlled by **chloropromazine** 0.05 mg/kg but must be used with caution in the presence of hypotension. Wrapping the patient in a wet sheet and blowing ambient air with a fan is another cooling method that may be effective.

   Dehydration is often a component of heat stroke, especially if the patient has been exercising and sweating for a prolonged period. Aggressive fluid resuscitation with **isotonic crystalloid** is indicated. Persistent hypotension may require inotropic support with agents such as **dobutamine,** which increases myocardial contractility while maintaining the peripheral vasodilation essential for heat dissipation.

   Urine output must be followed closely and maintained at >0.5 ml/kg/hr. Failure to maintain an adequate urine output with appropriate fluid resuscitation may indicate impending renal failure and should be managed with **furosemide** 1 mg/kg IV or **mannitol** 0.25 to 1 g/kg IV.

3. *Manage the complications of heat stroke.*

   Complications of heat stroke include dehydration and electrolyte abnormalities, acute renal failure, acute respiratory distress syndrome (ARDS), liver failure, rhabdomyolysis, seizures, and disseminated intravascular coagulation (DIC). Seizures may occur during the cooling phase. Screening for the above potential complications of heat stroke should include the following laboratory tests: CBC, electrolytes, BUN/Cr, PT/PTT, and urinalysis.

REFERENCES

Clowes G, O'Donnell T: Heat stroke, *N Engl J Med* 291:564-568, 1974.

Mellor MFA: Heat-induced illnesses. In Barkin RM: *Pediatric emergency medicine: concepts and clinical practice*, ed 2, St Louis, 1997, Mosby.

Sterner S: Summer heat illnesses, *Postgrad Med* 87:67-70, 1990.

Tek D, Olashaker JS: Heat illness, *Emerg Med Clin North Am* 10:299-310, 1992.

Thompson AE: Environmental emergencies. In Fleisher GR, Ludwig S, eds: *Textbook of pediatric emergency medicine*, ed 3, Baltimore, Williams & Wilkins, 1993, pp 810-815.

Vicario SJ, Okabajue R, Haltom T: Rapid cooling in classic heatstroke, *Am J Emerg Med* 4:394-398, 1986.

34. Electrical Injury

GUY L. UPSHAW

OBJECTIVES
1. Recognize the presentation of electrical injury.
2. Recognize and treat associated traumatic injuries.
3. Manage the complications of electrical injuries.

Brief Presenting History

A 10-year-old female has agonal respiration and burnt hands. Her mother reports, "I think she might have been shocked."

Initial Vital Signs

P 140, RR 8, BP 70/40.
If asked: T 37.2° C, estimated weight 30 kg.

Initial Physical Examination

General appearance: Poorly responsive, limp, school-age girl with odor of charred skin.
If asked:
- **Airway:** Patent, intact gag reflex.
- **Breathing:** Shallow, infrequent respirations that are symmetric, no retractions.
- **Circulation:** Tachycardic, no murmur, capillary refill time 5 seconds, distal pulses thready.
- HEENT: Normocephalic, atraumatic, pupils 6 mm, equal, sluggishly reactive.
- Abdomen: Soft, nondistended, bowel sounds present.
- Extremities: No deformities, mottled, cool.
- Skin: Charred and yellow-white lesions with surrounding erythema on right thumb and index finger and left palm.
- Neurologic: Poorly responsive to pain with some movement (withdrawal) of all extremities, brief eye opening to pain, and decreased tone.

Further History Given on Request

The mother left the patient doing dishes in the kitchen. Minutes later the lights and TV went out. The mother called the child and became concerned when she did not answer. The mother found the child on the floor beside the kitchen sink and noticed a burning smell in the air. She called 911 but did not wait for the ambulance. A police officer arrived to find an empty house and noted that the electricity was off and a charred electrical outlet and radio plug were next to the kitchen sink.
- Previously healthy, no chronic illnesses. No medications, NKDA.
- Tetanus toxoid at age 4.

Expected interventions	Complications
1. BVM-assisted ventilation with 100% O_2. In-line cervical spine immobilization. 2. Monitors (ECG and pulse oximeter). 3. Attempt IV access. Attempt femoral CVL. Laboratory tests: Rapid glucose, ABG, CBC, electrolytes, BUN/Cr, UA, urine myoglobin, cardiac enzymes. **Normal saline** or **Ringer's lactate** 20 ml/kg IV.	Patient vomits if no cricoid pressure applied. IV attempts unsuccessful.

Repeat Vital Signs

P 160, RR 0, BP 60/P, pulse oximeter 92%.

Progression

Patient is now apneic.

Expected interventions	Complications
1. Rapid sequence intubation. Preoxygenate with 100% O_2. No. 2 or 3 Mac/Miller laryngoscope blade. 6.5 uncuffed/6.0 cuffed ETT. Continued cricoid pressure until intubated. Place NG and end-tidal CO_2 monitor. Call for CXR to check ETT position. 2. Repeat **NS/RL** 20 ml/kg IV.	O_2 becomes disconnected. Pulse oximeter 80%. Vomits if no cricoid pressure.

Progression

Ventricular fibrillation on ECG monitor. (See p. 219 in Appendix E.)

Expected interventions	Complications
1. Palpate femoral pulse. 2. Defibrillate 1 to 2 J/kg asynchronous mode. 3. **Lidocaine** 1 mg/kg IV. See Cardiac Emergencies (p. 198) in Chapter 4.	No pulse palpated. Patient converts to sinus rhythm, pulse palpable.

Additional Potential Complications

1. Persistent ventricular fibrillation.
2. Seizure caused by neurologic injury from electric shock or hypoxia and acidosis.
3. Hypotension caused by blood loss from blunt thoracic or abdominal trauma. (May change mechanism of electrical injury to lightning strike or to a fall after receiving a shock while retrieving a kite from electrical wires.)

Disposition

ICU for continued management of electrical injury and complications, including trauma evaluation.

Discussion of Objectives

1. *Recognize the presentation of electrical injury.*

   Electrical injuries are associated with a wide range of complaints, from mild skin irritation and a "shock" sensation to full cardiopulmonary arrest. The extent of electrical injuries depends on the resistance and direction of electrical current through the patient's body, the type, frequency, and intensity of the current, and the duration of contact.

   In severe electrical injury the patient's skin often has electric current entrance and exit wounds, which may vary from mild superficial to full-thickness burns. High-voltage injuries such as lightning strikes, however, produce relatively small skin lesions and rarely lead to deep thermal injury because the exposure is instantaneous.

   Cardiac presentations include asystole (lightning) and ventricular fibrillation (high-voltage electrical), as well as supraventricular tachycardia, complete heart block, and ventricular extrasystoles. Patients may describe "crushing" chest pain resulting from direct myocardial injury. (See Cardiac Emergencies [p. 198] in Chapter 4.)

   Respiratory arrest may be caused by electric current injury to the medullary respiratory center or by tetanic contraction or paralysis of the diaphragm and chest wall muscles, or it may accompany primary cardiac arrest. Cardiac dysrhythmias may be induced by respiratory arrest.

   Symptoms of CNS injury and hypoxia include confusion, coma, seizures, and paralysis.

2. *Recognize and treat associated traumatic injuries.*

   Electrical injuries are associated with significant force. In the case of lightning strikes, up to 1 million volts may pass through a person. These huge forces offer great potential for traumatic injuries. Patients thrown by high voltage may have multiple traumatic injuries, including injury to the cervical spine. Patients who "lock on" to lower voltages are at risk for deep thermal injury. Patients with significant electrical exposures receive immobilization of the cervical spine and are evaluated in the same way as any other patient with multiple trauma. (See mock code 29, Multiple Blunt Trauma [p. 146] and Trauma [p. 203] in Chapter 4.)

3. *Manage the complications of electrical injuries.*

   Because of the multiple factors that determine the extent of electrical injuries and the direction of electrical flow through the body, all patients should be aggressively evaluated for life-threatening complications.

   Cardiopulmonary arrest is the most common cause of immediate death in severe electrical injury. Rapid assessment and support of the airway, breathing, and circulation are imperative.

Aggressive, prolonged resuscitation efforts are indicated because most patients with electrical injury are young and otherwise without preexisting cardiac disease and because extensive neurologic injury may lead to prolonged neurologic abnormalities such as impaired brainstem drive to breathe and anisocoria. Basic and advanced life support for respiratory failure and cardiac dysrhythmias is provided.

Rhabdomyolysis can be caused by severe electrical injury. The resultant renal myoglobin deposition can lead to acute tubular necrosis and renal failure. Emergency management requires aggressive hydration with **Ringer's lactate** or **normal saline** to maintain urine output at no less than 1 ml/kg/hr.

Additional Comments

1. **Succinylcholine** is contraindicated in electrically injured patients, who are prone to rhabdomyolysis and hyperkalemia.
2. Severe electrical shock often causes more internal injury than surface burns imply, so a high degree of suspicion for internal injury is warranted.
3. Other significant associated complications include large skin burns from ignited clothing and oral burns in small children from biting electrical cords.
4. Deep thermal injuries are associated with a high risk of infection. Tetanus toxoid should be given to patients who are not known to have been immunized within the past 5 years.

REFERENCES

Brown BJ, Gaasch WR: Electrical injuries and lightning, *Emerg Med Clin North Am* 10:211-229, 1992.

Emergency Cardiac Care Committee and Subcommittees, American Heart Association: Guidelines for cardiopulmonary resuscitation and emergency cardiac care: electrical shock and lightning strike, *JAMA* 268:2248-2249, 1992.

Fontanarosa PB: Electrical shock and lightning strike, *Ann Emerg Med* 22:378-387, 1993.

Hall ML, Sills RM: Electrical and lightning injuries. In Barkin RM: *Pediatric emergency medicine, concepts and clinical practice*, ed 2, St Louis, 1997, Mosby.

Thompson AE: Electrical injuries. In Fleisher GR, Ludwig S, eds: *Textbook of pediatric emergency medicine*, ed 3, Baltimore, 1993, Williams & Wilkins, pp 818-823.

35. Altitude Sickness—Pulmonary or Cerebral Edema
PAUL BOURESSA

OBJECTIVES
1. Recognize and formulate the differential diagnosis of respiratory distress.
2. Recognize the signs and symptoms of altitude or acute mountain sickness (AMS).
3. Manage altitude sickness and high-altitude pulmonary edema (HAPE).

Brief Presenting History

A 17-year-old male arrives at an emergency department in Aspen, Colorado, with fever, cough, and hemoptysis.

Initial Vital Signs

RR 38, HR 150, BP 120/70.
If asked: T 38.5° C (tympanic), estimated weight 70 kg.

Initial Physical Examination

General appearance: Moderate respiratory distress, anxious, and pale.
If asked:
- **Airway:** Patient breathing.
- **Breathing:** Intercostal retractions, crackles and wheezes more prominent on the right.
- **Circulation:** Tachycardia with normal S_1 and S_2, no murmurs, rubs, or gallops.
- Extremities: 1+ peripheral edema.
- Neurologic: Altered mental status with slight confusion, otherwise nonfocal.

Further History Given on Request

Previously healthy 17-year-old flew into Aspen from Boston 3 days ago for spring break. The last 2 days he has been complaining of insomnia, nausea, and loss of appetite. Today he went back-country skiing.
- NKDA.
- No medications, denies drug use, "two beers" last night.
- Past medical history negative.
- There is no history of trauma.

Expected interventions	Complications
1. 100% O_2. 2. Monitors (ECG and oximeter). 3. IV access, **normal saline** 20 ml/kg. 4. Laboratory tests: Rapid glucose, ABG, CBC, electrolytes, UA, urine toxicologic screen. 5. CXR, ECG. 6. Prepare for possible rapid sequence intubation.	Vomiting requires suction.

Repeat Vital Signs

RR 48, HR 150, BP 120/75.

Laboratory Findings

ABG: pH 7.48, Pco_2 28, Po_2 50, CBC: Hct 40, Plts 380k, Hgb 13.5, WBC 12,000, sodium 145, potassium 3.8, chloride 110, bicarbonate 20, BUN 28, creatinine 0.8, glucose 130.
UA: Trace positive for protein, otherwise negative with specific gravity 1.030.
Urine toxicologic screen: Negative.
CXR: Patchy alveolar and interstitial infiltrate R>L. Prominent pulmonary vessels with normal cardiac size. No pneumothorax.
ECG: RVH strain with sinus tachycardia.

Progression

Increased respiratory distress, worsening level of consciousness.

Expected interventions	Complications

1. Rapid sequence intubation.
    7.5 cuffed ETT.
    Miller/Mac blade no. 3.
    Midazolam 5 mg IV.
    Succinylcholine 100 mg IV.
    Cricoid pressure.
2. Place NG and end-tidal CO_2 monitor.
3. CXR for ETT position.
4. Arrange for transport to lower elevation.
	Initial intubation attempt fails, requires BVM with 100% O_2 and another attempt.
	Right mainstem intubation.
	
	Vomits if no cricoid pressure.

Progression

Bagging becomes more difficult. Acute desaturation to pulse oximetry reading of 75%. Patient becomes hypotensive.

Expected interventions	Complications

1. Auscultate chest.
   No breath sounds on right.
2. Needle right chest (see Thoracentesis [p. 12]
   in Chapter 2).
3. Place chest tube (see Thoracostomy Tube [p. 13]
   in Chapter 2).
	If tension pneumothorax not promptly
	addressed, progress to asystole.

◆

Additional Potential Complications

1. Cerebral edema with subsequent seizure.
2. Cardiac arrest caused by hypoxemia.

Disposition

After transport to lower elevation, hospital ward or ICU depending on response.

Discussion of Objectives

1. *Recognize and formulate the differential diagnosis of respiratory distress.*
   This patient displays obvious signs of respiratory distress with tachypnea and increased work of breathing. Oxygen saturation reveals hypoxia. The differential diagnosis includes reactive airways disease, infection (pneumonia or pneumonitis), pulmonary embolus, pneumothorax, congestive heart failure, trauma (hemothorax/pneumothorax, pulmonary contusion), foreign body aspiration, drug or alcohol ingestion, or other metabolic imbalance such as diabetic ketoacidosis (DKA).
2. *Recognize the signs and symptoms of altitude or acute mountain sickness (AMS).*
   AMS develops insidiously in young, healthy individuals, usually on the second to third day at altitude. Patients initially complain of appetite loss, nausea, insomnia, a "hung-over" feeling. The symptoms are exacerbated by rapid ascent to altitudes greater than 8000 feet, overexertion, dehydration, and use of alcohol. In some individuals AMS develops and then progresses to high-altitude pulmonary edema (HAPE) or high-altitude cerebral edema (HACE).
   Signs and symptoms of HAPE include dyspnea at rest, cough, frothy sputum, hemoptysis, cyanosis, tachypnea, tachycardia, and crackles on lung auscultation with normal cardiac findings. Patients may have fever, and physical examination findings that mimic pneumonia. Most important is historical information. The CXR typically shows bilateral diffuse fluffy infiltrates. There usually is evidence of pulmonary edema as well.
   Patients with HACE may have severe headache, vomiting, hallucinations, or seizures. Abnormal neurologic findings include ataxia, papilledema, and altered mental status. Again, historical data are the key to recognition. Other causes of altered mental status such as trauma or drug ingestion must be considered.

3. *Manage altitude sickness and high-altitude pulmonary edema.*

Prevention: Ascend slowly to allow acclimatization, avoid alcohol, avoid dehydration or overexertion, take **acetazolamide** for prophylaxis (respiratory stimulant and diuretic).

Treatment: The initial treatment is oxygen, but descent to a lower altitude is critical, especially in severe cases involving HAPE or HACE.

Additional supportive care includes hydration and analgesics. The efficacy of diuretics is controversial. **Dexamethasone** may be helpful in cases involving cerebral edema.

REFERENCES

Hackett PH, Rennie D: Rales, peripheral edema, retinal hemorrhage, and acute mountain sickness, *Am J Med* 67:214-220, 1979.

Johnson ST, Rock PB: Current concepts—acute mountain sickness, *N Engl J Med* 319:841-845, 1988.

Tso E: High-altitude illness, *Emerg Med Clin North Am* 10:231-247, 1992.

PREGNANCY-RELATED EMERGENCIES
36. Newborn Delivery and Resuscitation
DEBRA WEINER

OBJECTIVES
1. Recognize that two patients are involved.
2. Perform emergency delivery of a newborn.
3. Perform emergency resuscitation of a newborn.
4. Recognize the fetal and maternal factors that create risk to the newborn.

Brief Presenting History

A 15-year-old female has crampy, intermittent, abdominal pain. She is screaming with paroxysms or pain.

Initial Vital Signs

P120, BP 110/80, RR 24.
If asked: T 38.8° C (PO), estimated weight 50 kg.

Initial Physical Examination

General appearance: Uncomfortable, diaphoretic, obviously gravid, female.
If asked: cervix 10 cm dilated and 100% effaced. Head of neonate visible.

Further History Given on Request

- Mother denies knowledge of pregnancy (reportedly G_0P_0).
- No prenatal care.
- Date of last menstrual period uncertain but probably at least 6 or 7 months ago.
- No history of recent or current illness, abdominal trauma, or major medical problems.
- No medications, NKDA, denies cigarette smoking or drug use.

Expected interventions	Complications
1. Call appropriate services: obstetrics, neonatology departments.	
2. Delivery of newborn.	
Delivery of head.	
Suction nose and mouth at perineum.	Nuchal cord.
Delivery of body.	Shoulder dystocia.
Clamp and cut cord.	

Progression

Option 1: Full-term baby, pink, with grunting respirations.
Option 2: A very small, cyanotic baby delivered with minimal respiratory effort, minimal tone, no grimace.
Option 3: A large baby delivered through thick meconium, flexed, kicking, and slippery.

Vital Signs

Option 1: P 130, RR 40.
If asked: Weight 3.5 kg, 1-minute APGAR 7.
Option 2: P 40, RR 10.
If asked: Gestational age 28 weeks, 1000 g, 1-minute APGAR 3.
Option 3: P 100, RR 0.
If asked: Weight 4 kg, 1-minute APGAR 7.

Progression	Expected interventions
All options	
1. Transfer newborn to warming table.	
2. Suction mouth, nose.	Hypothermia if not properly dried and warmed.
3. Dry, remove wet towels.	
Option 1	
1. Stimulate, blow-by O_2.	
Option 2	
1. Stimulate, BVM ventilation with 100% O_2.	
2. Begin chest compressions.	
3. Intubate.	
Miller no. 0 blade.	Right mainstem intubation.
2.5 ETT.	Tube mishandled, falls out.
Option 3	
1. Intubate immediately to suction meconium.	
Miller No. 0 blade.	
3.5 ETT.	

Progression	Expected interventions	Complications
Option 1		
Baby improves with stimulation and O$_2$.	1. Keep baby warm. 2. Rapid glucose.	
Option 2		

Baby remains blue, no heartbeat.	1. Continue cardiac compressions.
	2. **Epinephrine** 1:10,000 via ETT 0.1 ml/kg diluted 1:1 in NS, repeat every 5 minutes.
	3. Rapid glucose.
	4. Umbilical vein catheterization (UVC).
	  Epinephrine 1:10,000, 0.1 ml/kg UVC.
	  D$_{10}$W 4 ml/kg UVC.
	  Normal saline 10 ml/kg UVC.
	  Laboratory tests: CBC, differential, platelets, blood culture, electrolytes, glucose, VBG.
		Rapid glucose 40.

	5. Needle the chest.	Pneumothorax from bag ventilations.
See Umbilical Vein Cannulation (p. 15) and Thoracentesis (p. 12) in Chapter 2.		
Option 3		
No respiratory effort after suctioning, loss of heart rate.	1. Reintubate. 2. Cardiac compressions. 3. Same as Option 2.	

Additional Potential Complications

1. Hypovolemia.
2. Multiple gestation.
3. Neonatal infection.
4. Postdelivery bleeding and hypotension in the mother.

Disposition

Option 1: Newborn nursery.

Options 2 and 3: NICU—replacement of umbilical venous catheter (UVC), placement of umbilical arterial catheter (UAC), urinalysis and urine culture, antibiotics, chest and abdomen films, vitamin K and ophthalmologic prophylaxis.

Discussion of Objectives

For general discussion of equipment and techniques for neonatal delivery and resuscitation refer to Chapters 1 and 2.

1. *Recognize that two patients are involved.*

   Early recognition that the patient is pregnant and that delivery is imminent is critical. Separate teams should attend to the mother and to the newborn when staff is available. Appropriate equipment for newborn delivery must be available.

2. *Perform emergency delivery of the newborn.*

   Pregnant patients with active contractions should be transported to appropriate facilities with labor and delivery wards whenever possible. However, if delivery is imminent, transfer is contraindicated. The mock code team should assess the condition of the mother and fetus and prepare for delivery. In the absence of continuous fetal monitoring the condition of the mother and pattern of labor are the best indicators of fetal condition.

3. *Emergency resuscitation of the newborn.*

   Resuscitation of the newborn, like any other pediatric patient, is based on attention to the ABCs. Because neonates have a large body surface area and are naked and wet after delivery, they are especially susceptible to hypothermia. Immediately after delivery the airway should be cleared with suction, oxygen should be applied, and the baby should be dried off with warm towels. A radiant heat source is used to keep the infant warm. After delivery of 15 to 30 seconds of BVM, chest compressions are begun if the heart rate is less than 60 or is 60 to 80 and not improving. After initial BVM ventilation with 100% oxygen the airway should be controlled by endotracheal (ET) intubation. Drugs of resuscitation (e.g., epinephrine, naloxone) may be administered via the ET tube. Poor tone and depressed respiratory effort may be related to maternal pain medications. The mother (or her obstetric care providers) should be questioned about peripartum medications, and she should be screened for increased risk of premature or complicated births.

4. *Recognize the fetal and maternal factors that create risk to the newborn.*

   Factors associated with premature delivery include:

   a. Maternal: Age ≤ 16 or ≥ 35, acute or chronic illness, abdominal trauma, poor nutrition, severe dehydration, cigarette smoking, drug use.

   b. Fetal: Intrauterine growth retardation (IUGR), multiple gestation, infection, anomalies, demise of the fetus.

   c. Placental: Previa, abruption, premature rupture of membranes, placentitis.

   d. Uterine: Cervical incompetence, uterine rupture, uterine abnormality, foreign body, chorioamnionitis, polyhydramnios.

   Factors associated with delayed response of newborn to resuscitation:

   a. Hypoxia and acidosis.

   b. Hypothermia.

   c. Hypoglycemia.

   d. Neurologic injury.

   See Neonatal Resuscitation (p. 204) in Chapter 4.

REFERENCES

Berry LM, Padbury JF: Newborn resuscitation. In Barkin RM: *Pediatric emergency medicine: concepts and clinical practice*, ed 2, St Louis, 1997, Mosby.

Jain L, Vidyasagar D: Controversies in neonatal resuscitation, *Pediatr Ann* 25:540-545, 1995.

Schafermeyer RW: Neonatal resuscitation. In Fleisher GR, Ludwig S, eds: *Textbook of pediatric emergency medicine*, ed 3, Baltimore, 1993, Williams & Wilkins, pp 32-43.

37. Pregnancy with Vaginal Bleeding

DEBRA WEINER

OBJECTIVES

1. Recognize that two patients are involved.
2. Manage the pregnant patient with obstetric bleeding and precipitous delivery.
3. Recognize maternal conditions associated with and resulting from obstetric bleeding.

Brief Presenting History

An obese 15-year-old female has abdominal pain and vaginal bleeding.

Initial Vital Signs

P 120, BP 110/80, RR 24.
If asked: T 38.8° C (PO), estimated weight 85 kg.

Initial Physical Examination

General appearance: Alert, anxious, obese, and gravid female.
Abdomen: Bowel sounds present, soft, unable to palpate liver, spleen, or masses.
Option 1: (Mild abruption) Pain crampy and intermittent, abdomen mildly tender diffusely.
If asked: Cervix is dilated to 10 cm and 100% effaced. Head of neonate is intermittently visible. Small gushes of dark blood with clots per vagina.
Option 2: (Moderate abruption) Pain crampy and intermittent, abdomen moderately tender throughout.
Option 3: (Severe abruption) Pain crampy and intermittent, abdomen severely tender with vaginal bleeding.
Options 2 and 3:
If asked: Cervix is dilated to 10 cm and 100% effaced. Head of neonate is intermittently visible. Moderate to severe vaginal bleeding, dark blood with clots (abruption with vaginal bleeding).

Further History Given on Request

Patient denies knowledge of pregnancy and has had no prenatal care. Date of last menstrual period uncertain but probably at least 6 or 7 months ago. Denies recent or current illness.

- No previous pregnancies.
- No history of abdominal trauma.
- Denies major medical problems, medications, tobacco or drug use.
- NKDA.

Expected interventions	Complications
1. Call appropriate services: obstetrics, neonatology departments. 2. ECG monitor, pulse oximeter. 3. 100% oxygen. 4. Two large-bore IVs. **NS** 20 ml/kg IV. Call for **O-negative blood**. 5. Laboratory tests: type and cross 4 units, CBC, blood culture, Coombs, VDRL, toxicologic screen. 6. Deliver infant (see mock code 36, Newborn Delivery and Resuscitation, p. 179). 7. Deliver placenta. 8. Empiric antibiotics.	If digital vaginal examination performed, hemorrhage and significant hypotension result.

Progression	Expected interventions	Complications
Option 1 No maternal distress. P 140, BP 90/60, RR 18.	1. Supportive care and monitoring. 2. Resuscitate infant (2nd team).	Premature delivery.
Option 2 Mild hypovolemia. P 160, BP 70/P, RR 12. Capillary refill time 3 to 4 seconds.	1. Repeat **normal saline** 20 ml/kg IV. 2. Resuscitate infant (second team). 3. Colloid, **5% albumin,** or **O-negative blood.**	Premature delivery. Persistent hypovolemia.
Option 3 Altered mental status, peripheral pulses weak, extremities cool, P 180, BP 50/P, RR 6.	1. Repeat **normal saline** 20 ml/kg IV. 2. Resuscitate infant (second team). 3. Colloid, **5% albumin,** or **O-negative blood.** 4. Rapid sequence intubation. Miller or Mac no. 3 blade, 7 to 8 ETT. **Midazolam** 5 mg IV. **Succinylcholine** 100 mg IV or **vecuronium** 10 mg IV. Cricoid pressure. 5. Place NG and end-tidal CO_2 monitor. 6. CXR for ETT position. 7. Foley catheter.	Premature delivery. Persistent hypovolemia, poor respiratory effort. Right mainstem intubation. Tube falls out if not properly taped and handled. Vomits if no cricoid pressure or NG tube.

Additional Potential Complications

1. Full-term arrest in infant caused by hypoxia in the perinatal period.
2. Multiple gestation.
3. Disseminated intravascular coagulation (DIC) in mother, necessitating resuscitation with fresh frozen plasma (FFP) or cryoprecipitate.

Disposition

Option 1: Obstetrics ward or ICU.
Option 2 or 3: ICU or OR for exploration of vaginal bleeding.

Discussion of Objectives

1. *Recognize that two patients are involved.*
   Early recognition that the patient is pregnant and that delivery is imminent is critical. Separate teams should attend to the mother and to the newborn. Each team should ideally consist of at least two health care professionals with at least one physician per team.
   Appropriate equipment must be available for adult and infant resuscitation. (For list of equipment required see p. 4 in Chapter 1.)
2. *Manage the pregnant patient with obstetric bleeding and precipitous delivery (Box 3-1).*
   History and physical should be directed at identifying type and degree of bleeding. Attempt to determine gestational age of fetus, history of maternal conditions that predispose to obstetric bleeding, fetal position, heart rate, uterine contractions, character, quantity, and site of bleeding, pain.
   Do not perform vaginal or rectal examination if there is concern that bleeding may be due to placenta previa, placental abruption, or rupture of the uterus, since this may induce severe hemorrhage. Emergency delivery is indicated when delivery is imminent or when the amount of bleeding is a threat to maternal or fetal well-being.
3. *Recognize maternal conditions associated with and resulting from obstetric bleeding.*
   Maternal conditions predisposing to obstetric bleeding and precipitous preterm delivery include hypertension, infection, and injury secondary to trauma.
   Maternal conditions resulting from obstetric bleeding and precipitous preterm delivery include hypovolemic shock, disseminated intravascular coagulation, respiratory failure, cardiac arrest, renal failure.

BOX 3-1

PLACENTAL CAUSES OF BLEEDING

Placental Abruption

Premature separation of placenta from uterus

Two types of bleeding possible:

1. External hemorrhage secondary to peripheral separation of placenta with egress of blood through cervix and vagina
2. Concealed hemorrhage secondary to bleeding between placenta and uterus with trapping of blood retroplacentally without vaginal bleeding

Mild abruption: Vaginal bleeding scant to moderate, dark, blood with mild lower abdominal discomfort; mother is hemodynamically stable, blood loss is minimal, and no fetal distress exists.

Moderate abruption: Vaginal bleeding is absent if hemorrhage is concealed, but moderate, continuous uterine pain is present. Pain may be more severe if concealed hemorrhage; minimal maternal risk despite fetal distress with possible fetal demise.

Severe abruption: Vaginal bleeding ranges from absent to severe. Continuous severe stabbing uterine pain, usually with maternal shock, often DIC, renal failure, severe fetal distress or demise. Incidence: 1 in 100 to 120. It usually occurs after 28th week of gestation. Increased incidence with toxemia of pregnancy, maternal hypertension, renal disease, trauma, and cocaine use.

Placenta Previa

Placenta is implanted in the lower pole of uterus near or over the os.
Painless bleeding secondary to separation of placenta from uterus.
Incidence 1 in 200; 80% in multiparous women, increased in women over age 35.
Usually abnormal fetal position.
May be associated with multiple gestation.

Abortion or Threatened Abortion

More likely if bleeding is with cramping.

Bloody Show

Painless discharge of blood and mucus before delivery.

Ruptured Uterus

Pain and vaginal or concealed bleeding.
Incidence: 1 in 100 women previously delivered by cesarean section.

Ruptured Vasa Previa

Painless vaginal bleeding without contractions, but with fetal distress.
Occurs rarely.

Additional Comments

1. Leukocystosis with WBC up to 30,000/mm^3 is normal during labor and delivery.
2. A fourth option that may be used is abruption with retroplacental bleeding. This entity may be manifested as constant, sharp abdominal pain and scant vaginal bleeding.
3. See Neonatal Resuscitation (p. 204) in Chapter 4.

REFERENCES

Ammerman S, Shafer M, Snyder D: Ectopic pregnancy in adolescents: a clinical review for pediatricians, *J Pediatr* 117:677-686, 1990.

Hockberger RS: Ectopic pregnancy, *Emerg Clin North Am* 5:481-493, 1987.

4 Initial Approaches

This chapter summarizes some of the essential concepts illustrated in Chapter 3. It discusses the basic approaches and algorithms the practitioner might use, given certain common presenting problems such as respiratory distress, asystole, coma, and increased intracranial pressure, as well as their potential etiologies. This chapter is intended as a quick summary only. References are offered for more in-depth review.

1. INITIAL APPROACH TO AIRWAY OBSTRUCTION

MARK G. ROBACK

1. The airway is proportionately smaller in children and infants than in adults, whereas the tongue is proportionately larger relative to the oropharynx.
2. The narrowest portion of the airway in adults is the glottic inlet. In infants and children less than approximately 8 years of age the narrowest part is below the level of the cords.
3. Pediatric vocal cords are more anteriorly positioned.
4. Airway obstruction in the pediatric airway can occur with minimal insult such as swelling, secretions, positioning, and decreased tone.

History

Consider common causes of airway obstruction such as:
1. Foreign body aspiration.
2. Infection: Viral (croup), bacterial (epiglottitis), or soft tissue infections of the pharynx.
3. Trauma.
4. Conditions of decreased tone, postictal state, or neuromuscular disease.
5. Conditions of increased secretions and decreased ability to clear secretions.

Physical Examination

Look for signs of respiratory insufficiency.
1. General appearance: Level of consciousness, work of breathing.
2. Airway: Ability to move air, audible stridor.
3. Chest: Respiratory rate, inspiratory/expiratory phase ratio, presence of retractions, or evidence of other accessory muscle use.
4. Auscultation: Listen over the airway for air entry, stridor, or wheeze.
5. Cardiac: Perfusion, capillary refill, skin color, presence of mottling, character of heart tones and pulses.

Resuscitation

1. 100% Oxygen.
2. Positioning: Place head in midline, jaw thrust, chin lift and head tilt (contraindicated in trauma).
3. Suction: Clear airway of secretions, vomitus, and foreign bodies as indicated.
4. Insert oral or nasal airways.
5. Assist with bag-valve-mask ventilation as needed.
6. Intubate the trachea if above is not adequate.
7. Consider alternative airway techniques such as placement of a surgical airway (see Cricothyrotomy in Chapter 2) if endotracheal intubation is contraindicated or unsuccessful.

REFERENCES

American Heart Association and American Association of Pediatrics: Airway and ventilation. In *Textbook of pediatric advanced life support*, 1994.

2. INITIAL APPROACH TO RESPIRATORY DISTRESS

MARK G. ROBACK

History

Consider common causes of respiratory distress such as:

1. Pulmonary.
    a. Upper airway obstruction, foreign body, infection, congenital anomaly.
    b. Asthma, bronchiolitis.
    c. Pneumonia.
    d. Cystic fibrosis.
2. Sepsis.
3. Cardiac.
    a. Congenital: Ductal-dependent lesions, other causes of congested heart failure.
    b. Acquired: Cardiomyopathies.
4. Metabolic acidosis.
    a. Gastroenteritis and dehydration.
    b. Diabetic ketoacidosis.
    c. Ingestions, including salicylates and alcohols.
    d. Inborn errors of metabolism.
5. Neurologic.
    a. Trauma.
    b. CNS infection.
    c. Status epilepticus.
    d. Neuromuscular disease.

Physical Examination

1. ABCs.
2. General appearance: Look for signs of acute respiratory distress such as agitation, air hunger, and posture (sniffing position).
3. Respiratory examination: Auscultate breath sounds (decreased, symmetric), and note presence of stridor, wheezing, and crackles, as well as accessory muscle use.
4. Cardiac examination: Assess color and perfusion; auscultate heart sounds for murmurs, gallop, and rub; palpate quality of pulses.
5. Neurologic examination: Assess level of consciousness.
6. Abdomen: Look for hepatomegaly.
7. Pulse oximetry, ABG, and CXR may be helpful.

Resuscitation

1. Administration of 100% oxygen is rarely contraindicated in children and therefore is a good first step.
2. Use the history and physical examination to narrow the pathogenesis, and proceed accordingly.
3. If the patient is apneic, initiate positive-pressure ventilations with bag-valve-mask and prepare to intubate.
4. If primary pulmonary disease is suspected, differentiate between upper or lower airway obstruction and parenchymal disease.
5. Treatment of nonpulmonary causes of respiratory distress should be directed toward the underlying etiology.

REFERENCES

Baren JM, Seidel JS: Emergency management of respiratory distress and failure. In Barkin RM: *Pediatric emergency medicine: concepts and clinical practice*, ed 2, St Louis, 1997, Mosby.

Thompson AE: Respiratory distress. In Fleisher GR, Ludwig S, eds: *Textbook of pediatric emergency medicine*, ed 3, Baltimore, 1993, Williams & Wilkins, pp 450-455.

3. INITIAL APPROACH TO SHOCK

RICHARD BACHUR

History

Differentiate the common types of shock:
1. Hypovolemic: Intravascular volume loss; water losses from diarrhea and vomiting; hemorrhage; plasma losses (burns, hypoproteinemia).
2. Distributive: Includes sepsis, anaphylaxis, and spinal shock.
3. Cardiogenic: Congestive heart failure of any etiology. Also:
   a. Myocardial dysfunction (myocarditis, cardiomyopathy, ischemia, acidosis).
   b. Pericardial (tamponade, constrictive pericarditis).
   c. Outflow tract obstruction (coarctation of the aorta, pulmonary embolus).
   d. Dysrhythmias (supraventricular tachycardia, heart block).

Physical Examination

Differentiate the causes of shock.

1. ABCs.
2. General appearance: Acute distress, level of consciousness.
3. Skin: Color, presence of rashes, edema.
4. Respiratory examination: Breath sounds (decreased, symmetric), stridor, wheezing, crackles, accessory muscle use.
5. Cardiac examination: Heart sounds, murmurs, gallop, rub, peripheral perfusion, pulses.
6. Abdomen: Enlarged liver or spleen.
7. Pulse oximeter, ABG, and CXR may be helpful.

Note: Early indicators of shock include tachycardia, prolonged capillary refill time, and decreased urine output. Low blood pressure is a *late* finding in shock.

Resuscitation

1. Secure airway, and administer 100% oxygen.
2. Start bag-valve-mask ventilation. Intubate early (before complete cardiopulmonary collapse).
3. Provide vascular access.
   a. Begin attempts with peripheral veins.
   b. After 90 seconds of elapsed time or two failed attempts, proceed to intraosseous or central venous access.
   c. Two or more sites of access are desirable.
   d. Control hemorrhage if present.
4. Order laboratory tests. Hematocrit, rapid serum glucose, and blood type and screen are the most important. Other laboratory tests to consider: ABG, CBC, electrolytes with BUN/Cr, blood culture, PT/PTT.
5. Initiate monitoring: Cardiac, pulse oximeter, temperature, indwelling urine catheter (for monitoring urine output).
6. Administer fluids.
   a. Isotonic crystalloid 20 ml/kg, monitor response, repeat if response insufficient.
   b. In cases of trauma or known hemorrhage, if patient shows poor response to isotonic crystalloid bolus of 20 ml/kg given twice, administer blood (O-negative until blood can be typed or matched).
   c. *Fluid boluses are contraindicated in congestive heart failure (CHF)*; however, do not withhold fluids unless a *strong* suspicion of CHF (gallop, jugular venous distention, hepatomegaly, crackles, cardiomegaly) exists.
7. Assess response to fluid bolus. Positive responses include improved perfusion, decreased heart rate, and increased blood pressure. If poor or no response, give *second* 20 ml/kg bolus of isotonic crystalloid; at the same time, plan for the addition of pressors or use of colloid (**5% albumin** or blood) if no response to the second 20 ml/kg bolus is seen.
8. Vasoconstrictors and inotropes: First-line drugs administered as a continuous IV infusion.
   a. **Epinephrine** (begin at 0.1 µg/kg/min) and
   b. **Dopamine** (begin at 10 µg/kg/min).

9. Consider:
   a. Empiric antibiotics when sepsis is suspected.
   b. CXR if trauma or concern about tension pneumothorax, pericardial tamponade, or congestive heart failure.
   c. Surgical consult if concern about trauma.
10. In cases of trauma: Continue to replace volume with blood (administer fresh frozen plasma or platelets or both if a coagulopathy is present or for every 4 units of packed red blood cells administered).
11. In cardiogenic shock, inotropes may be required. Administer **dobutamine** (begin at 10 μg/kg/min).
12. Continue to monitor and reassess (heart rate, blood pressure, perfusion, urine output, mental status, acid-base status).

Other Modalities, Interventions, and Considerations

1. Insert an arterial catheter, especially if the patient is receiving pressors.
2. Central venous pressure (CVP) monitoring is helpful for assessing response to fluids, especially if concerns about a cardiac component to the shock state exist (can also obtain samples for mixed-venous oxygen measurement).
3. Consider steroids only when adrenal suppression is suspected, as in steroid dependency from chronic use or congenital adrenal hyperplasia. Steroids are otherwise not indicated in the management of shock.
4. Prostaglandins may help infants in shock caused by ductal-dependent heart disease.
5. Look for and correct disseminated intravascular coagulopathy (DIC) in association with shock.
6. Correct acidosis if severe or if no improvement occurs after initial interventions.

REFERENCES

Bell LM: Shock. In Fleisher GR, Ludwig S, eds: *Textbook of pediatric emergency medicine*, ed 3, Baltimore, 1993, Williams & Wilkins, pp 44-54.
Hazinksi MF, Barkin RM: Shock. In Barkin RM: *Pediatric emergency medicine, concepts and clinical practice*, ed 2, St Louis, 1997, Mosby.

4. INITIAL APPROACH TO NEUROLOGIC EMERGENCIES
A. Altered Mental Status

MARK G. ROBACK

History

Consider the common causes of altered mental status:

1. Trauma: Head injury, mass lesion (blood), diffuse axonal injury, increased intracranial pressure, shaken baby syndrome.
2. Ingestion and intoxication: Many drugs and poisons.

3. CNS infections: Meningitis, encephalitis, abscess.
4. Shock: Septic, cardiogenic, hypovolemic.
5. Hypoxia and hypercapnia: Airway edema, inflammation, foreign body, cystic fibrosis.
6. Metabolic: Hypoglycemia, diabetic ketoacidosis, electrolyte derangements, inborn errors of metabolism.
7. Postictal state: Seizure and anticonvulsant levels.
8. Intracranial mass: Tumor, nontraumatic bleeding, abscess.
9. Hepatic encephalopathy, Reye's syndrome.
10. Hypothermia.
11. Intussusception.
12. Psychiatric or behavioral disorders.

Physical Examination

1. Attention to the ABCs.
2. Respiratory: Rate and pattern of breathing, quality of air entry, breath sounds.
3. Cardiac: Rate, peripheral perfusion, pulses.
4. Neurologic: Level of consciousness, focal neurologic findings, pupillary response, fundoscopic examination, tone.
5. Head and skin: Evidence of trauma, neck rigidity.

Resuscitation

Resuscitation is directed toward the underlying cause. If the history and physical examination do not yield a likely diagnosis, the following therapy and laboratory data may be helpful:

1. 100% Oxygen.
2. Rapid serum glucose determination.
3. ECG and pulse oximetry readings.
4. ABG.
5. Electrolytes, CBC, ammonia.
6. Toxicologic screen, acetaminophen and aspirin levels.

Empiric Medications To Be Considered

1. **Dextrose** 0.25 to 0.5 g/kg IV delivered as 1 to 2 ml/kg $D_{25}W$.
2. **Thiamine** 50 to 100 mg IV. When dextrose is administered to adolescents with chronic alcoholism or malnutrition, thiamine also should be given because dextrose infusion may precipitate symptoms of Wernicke's encephalopathy because of thiamine deficiency. Typically not required for infants and young children.
3. **Naloxone** 0.1 mg/kg IV/IM/ETT (approximately 1 mg for young children, 2 mg for school-children and older). Repeat every 2 to 5 minutes as needed to a total dose of 10 to 20 mg. Be aware that naloxone can precipitate an abstinence syndrome in patients with chronic narcotic use.
4. **Flumazenil**.
   a. Infant (up to 6 months old): 0.02 mg/kg (up to 0.2 mg) IV/IM over 15 seconds. May be repeated every 45 seconds to a maximum dose of 1 mg in the first hour.

  b. Pediatric (over 6 months)/adult: 0.2 mg IV/IM over 15 seconds, followed 45 seconds later by 0.3 mg, followed 45 seconds later by 0.5 mg to a maximum dose of 3 mg in the first hour. May be given as a continuous IV infusion.

  c. Indications: May be useful in patients with known or suspected benzodiazepine or mixed drug overdose who display coma, respiratory depression, or profound lethargy.

  d. Contraindications: Absolutely contraindicated in any patient with known or suspected overdose of any of the cyclic antidepressants, in any patient with seizure acutely treated with benzodiazepines, and in any patient with long-term benzodiazepine treatment for a seizure disorder.

REFERENCES

Fuchs SM et al: Neurologic disorders. In Barkin RM: *Pediatric emergency medicine: concepts and clinical practice*, ed 2, St Louis, 1997, Mosby.

Packer RJ, Berman PH: Coma. In Fleisher GR, Ludwig S, eds: *Textbook of pediatric emergency medicine*, ed 3, Baltimore, 1993, Williams & Wilkins, pp 122-134.

B. Seizures

RICHARD BACHUR

History

Consider the common causes of seizure:

1. Epilepsy: Subtherapeutic anticonvulsant levels or breakthrough seizures caused by intercurrent illness.
2. Head trauma: With or without intracranial bleeding, consider shaken baby syndrome.
3. Infectious: Meningitis, encephalitis, abscess.
4. Metabolic: Hypoglycemia, hyponatremia, hypocalcemia, hypomagnesemia, hypophosphatemia, hypernatremia.
5. Toxicologic: Ingestions.
6. Hypoxia: Including carbon monoxide poisoning.
7. Hypertensive crisis.
8. Inflammatory: Hemolytic uremic syndrome (HUS), systemic lupus erythematosus (SLE), vasculitides.
9. Tumor or other mass lesions that lead to increased intracranial pressure (ICP).
10. Vascular: Stroke, arteriovenous malformation (AVM), hemorrhage with idiopathic thrombocytopenia (ITP) or hemophilia.

Physical Examination

1. Attention to the ABCs.
2. Respiratory: Rate and pattern of breathing, quality of air entry, breath sounds.
3. Cardiac: Rate, peripheral perfusion, pulses.
4. Neurologic: Level of consciousness, focal findings, pupillary response, fundoscopic examination, tone, reflexes.
5. Head: Evidence of trauma, quality of anterior fontanel if age appropriate.
6. Neck: Rigidity.

Resuscitation

1. Oxygen, secure airway (consider jaw thrust, airway adjuncts, suctioning of secretions).
2. Cervical spine precautions if concern about trauma exists.
3. Laboratory tests to be considered, depending on presentation: Rapid serum glucose, electrolytes, calcium, phosphorus, magnesium, CBC, blood culture, ABG, toxicologic screen, and ammonia. If hypoglycemia exists, consider more extensive metabolic laboratory evaluation.
4. Anticonvulsants.
   a. First line, benzodiazepines.
      Lorazepam: 0.05 to 0.1 mg/kg IV.
      Diazepam: 0.1 to 0.3 mg/kg IV; 0.3 to 0.5 mg/kg PR.
   b. Second line.
      Phenytoin: 10 to 20 mg/kg (in normal saline administered not faster than 1 mg/kg/min).
      Phenobarbitol: 10 to 20 mg/kg IV or IM.
   c. Third line.
      Paraldehyde 300 mg/kg/dose (with equal volume of corn oil) PR. (Many hospital pharmacies no longer stock paraldehyde.)
   Note: Most anticonvulsants given in an acute case of status epilepticus are respiratory suppressive. The practitioner must always be prepared to control the airway and assist breathing when treating acute seizures.
5. Additional therapies and diagnostic measures to be considered.
   a. Antibiotics when sepsis or CNS infection is suspected.
   b. **Pyridoxine** 100 mg IV empirically for infants with first-time seizures and no obvious etiology.
   c. CT scan of the head if an intracranial lesion is suspected.

REFERENCES

Fuchs SM et al: Neurologic disorders. In Barkin RM: *Pediatric emergency medicine: concepts and clinical practice*, ed 2, St Louis, 1997, Mosby.

Packer RJ, Berman PH: Neurologic emergencies. In Fleisher GR, Ludwig S, eds: *Textbook of pediatric emergency medicine*, ed 3, Baltimore, 1993, Williams & Wilkins, pp 573-581.

C. Increased Intracranial Pressure

MARK G. ROBACK

History

Consider the common causes of increased intracranial pressure (ICP):

1. Trauma: Intracranial bleeding, diffuse swelling.
2. Infection: Meningitis, encephalitis, cerebral abscess.
3. Tumor or other intracranial mass.
4. Nontraumatic bleeding: Ruptured aneurysm or AVM.
5. Nontraumatic cerebral edema: Metabolic fluid shifts.

Physical Examination

1. ABCs.
2. Respiratory: Rate and pattern of breathing, quality of air entry, breath sounds.
3. Cardiac: Rate, perfusion, pulses.
4. Neurologic: Level of consciousness, fundoscopic exam.
   a. Focal neurologic findings: Third nerve, motor, and postural abnormalities.
   b. Ophthalmoplegia and Cushing's triad (bradycardia, hypertension, and abnormal respiratory pattern) are typically *late* findings indicative of impending brainstem herniation or chronic increased ICP.

Resuscitation

The management goal is *to lower ICP while maintaining cerebral perfusion pressure.*

$$CPP = MAP - ICP$$

CPP = cerebral perfusion pressure.

MAP = mean arterial pressure.

ICP = intracranial pressure.

1. Aggressively support blood pressure with volume (**5% albumin** if crystalloid is ineffective).
2. Intubate and hyperventilate: P_{CO_2} approximately 30 to 35 (do *not* overventilate).
3. Mannitol diuresis: Goal is to achieve serum osmolality of 305 to 315 mmol/kg (*only* if peripheral perfusion is adequate). Place a Foley catheter to monitor urine output.
4. Control seizures: If CT shows blood in parenchyma, consider empiric treatment with **phenytoin** 10 to 20 mg/kg IV delivered at a rate not to exceed 1 mg/kg/min. Given too rapidly, infusion of dilantin may lead to cardiovascular collapse.
5. **Dexamethasone** is indicated only for the treatment of intracranial tumors and in spinal cord trauma.

REFERENCES

Bruce DA: Neurosurgical emergencies. In Fleisher GR, Ludwig S, eds: *Textbook of pediatric emergency medicine,* ed 3, Baltimore, 1993, Williams & Wilkins, pp 1410-1416.

Bruce, DA: Head trauma. In Fleisher GR, Ludwig S, eds: *Textbook of pediatric emergency medicine,* ed 3, Baltimore, 1993, Williams & Wilkins, pp 1102-1112.

5. INITIAL APPROACH TO CARDIAC EMERGENCIES
A. Asystole

RICHARD BACHUR

Remember to treat the patient, *not* the monitor. If the monitor rhythm is asystole, be sure to:

1. Check for pulses.
2. Check placement of leads.
3. Confirm in two different leads to be sure that the rhythm is not fine ventricular fibrillation.
4. If the patient does not have pulses, do not delay the initiation of CPR while confirming rhythm.

History

Primary cardiac arrest or asystole is uncommon in pediatrics. In most pediatric patients asystole is a result of respiratory failure. The history is directed at determining the cause of asystole.

Physical Examination

Determine that the patient is without a pulse or heart rate and proceed directly to resuscitation.

Resuscitation

1. Secure the airway and administer 100% oxygen.
2. Ventilate (bag-valve-mask) immediately. Intubate early in the course.
3. If pulses are absent, initiate chest compressions.
   a. Obtain IV or IO access.
   b. Laboratory tests: Rapid serum glucose, ABG, CBC, and electrolytes.
4. **Epinephrine** 0.01 mg/kg (0.1 ml/kg of 1:10,000) IV/IO. If given via ETT, 0.1 mg/kg (10 times the usual dose except in newborns).
   a. Second and subsequent doses of epinephrine should be 10 times the initial dose, so-called high-dose epi 0.1 mg/kg (0.1 ml/kg, 1:1000).
   b. Repeat every 3 minutes followed by a fluid flush.
   c. A continuous IV infusion may be required, 0.1 to 1 μg/kg/min.
5. Continue to check for pulses or rhythm change every 5 minutes. If rhythm changes to bradycardia, ventricular tachycardia, or ventricular fibrillation, continue along those specific algorithms.
6. Consider attempt at defibrillation at 2 J/kg asynchronous mode (some clinicians advocate an attempt at defibrillation after 5 minutes or more of CPR, since fine ventricular fibrillation may not have been recognized).

Note: Asystole is the most common rhythm in pediatric cardiopulmonary arrest and usually is the result of a prolonged arrest. No effective therapy exists except in special circumstances such as hypothermia or hyperkalemia.

REFERENCES

Ludwig S, Kettrick RG: Resuscitation—pediatric basic and advanced life support. In Fleisher GR, Ludwig S, eds: *Textbook of pediatric emergency medicine*, ed 3, Baltimore, 1993, Williams & Wilkins, p 26.

Seidel JS: Cardiopulmonary resuscitation. In Barkin RM: *Pediatric emergency medicine: concepts and clinical practice*, ed 2, St Louis, 1997, Mosby.

B. Bradycardia

RICHARD BACHUR

History

Determine the possible etiologies of bradycardia. *Bradycardia in pediatrics is usually the result of respiratory failure.*

1. Sinus bradycardia: Increased vagal tone, increased intracranial pressure, drugs, hypothyroidism, hypoxia, acidosis.
2. Conduction defects.
   a. Congenital.
   b. Acquired: Postsurgical, myocarditis, systemic lupus erythematosus, rheumatic fever, infarction.
   c. Drug induced.
   d. Metabolic: Severe acidosis, hyperkalemia, hypercalcemia, hypermagnesemia, hypoglycemia.

Physical Examination

Focus on the ABCs and determine perfusion to end organs.

1. **Airway**: Assess patency of airway.
2. **Breathing**: Assess respiratory effort, air entry, accessory muscle use, and breath sounds.
3. **Cardiovascular**: Observe skin color. Check perfusion by determining capillary refill time, palpate pulses for quality, and auscultate heart sounds for loudness, rhythm, or extra sounds such as murmurs, gallops, rubs, or clicks.
4. Disability: Assess level of consciousness.

Resuscitation

1. Establish the airway, and administer 100% oxygen.
2. Hyperventilate, with bag-valve-mask assistance as needed.
3. Check for pulses. If absent, begin chest compressions.
   a. Establish bradycardia: Must determine if cardiovascular signs (e.g., hypotension) are present before deciding how to treat.
   b. Slow rhythms may or may not be associated with p-waves and may be narrow or wide complex based on pacemaker site and cause of bradycardia.
   c. Obtain IV access (coincidentally order routine laboratory tests, including rapid serum glucose, ABG, electrolytes, calcium, and magnesium).
4. If a primary conduction defect (e.g., heart block—congenital, postsurgical, nonpostsurgical acquired) is suspected, give:
   a. **Atropine** 0.02 mg/kg IV (minimum dose 0.1 mg). (*Note:* Use of atropine below the minimum recommended dose may lead to paradoxical bradycardia.) If no response is observed,
   b. **Epinephrine** 0.01 mg/kg (0.1 ml/kg, 1:10,000) IV, or begin
   c. **Isoproterenol** 0.1 μg/kg/min continuous IV infusion.
   External or transvenous pacing should also be considered. Rule out metabolic causes. Advance the isoproterenol drip until the desired heart rate response is achieved. If the heart rate responds but shock persists, consider volume resuscitation and alpha-agonists.

5. If hypoxic insult is suspected, give **epinephrine** 0.01 mg/kg IV or IO/ETT initially followed by atropine and pacing. Continue ventilation with 100% oxygen, and treat metabolic abnormalities. If the heart rate responds and shock persists, consider volume resuscitation and alpha-agonists.

REFERENCES

Ludwig S, Kettrick RG: Resuscitation—pediatric basic and advanced life support. In Fleisher GR, Ludwig S, eds: *Textbook of pediatric emergency medicine*, ed 3, Baltimore, 1993, Williams & Wilkins, pp 26-27.

C. Tachycardia

ANDREW ATZ

History

Determine which causes of tachycardia are possible.
1. Automatic tachycardia: "Warmup and cooldown" onset and termination.
   a. Sinus tachycardia: Dehydration, fever, pain, stress, medicines, ingestions.
   b. Ectopic atrial tachycardia.
   c. Junctional ectopic tachycardia.
2. Reentrant tachycardia: Abrupt onset and termination.
   a. Accessory pathway (Wolff-Parkinson-White syndrome, concealed pathway).
3. Atrial flutter or fibrillation.
4. Ventricular tachycardia.

Physical Examination

Focus on the ABCs and determine perfusion to end organs.
1. **Airway**: Assess patency of the airway.
2. **Breathing**: Assess respiratory effort, air entry, accessory muscle use, and breath sounds.
3. **Cardiovascular**: Observe skin color. Check perfusion by determining capillary refill time, palpate pulses for quality, and auscultate heart sounds for loudness, rhythm, or extra sounds such as murmurs, gallops, rubs, or clicks.
4. Disability: Assess level of consciousness.

Resuscitation

1. Establish the airway. Administer 100% oxygen.
2. Provide bag-valve-mask–assisted ventilation as needed.
3. If no pulse is appreciated, begin CPR.
4. *Always obtain a 12-lead ECG. A rhythm strip is not sufficient.*
5. Observe heart rate response to treatment of symptoms such as an antipyretic in fever, volume resuscitation in dehydration, or analgesics for pain control. Automatic tachycardias slow when catecholamines are reduced, whereas reentrant rhythms remain constant.

6. Treatment for specific tachycardias.

   a. Any patient with a reentrant tachycardia who is unresponsive or otherwise hemodynamically unstable should receive immediate synchronized cardioversion 0.5 to 1 J/kg.

   b. Patients who are clinically stable and alert and have a perfusing blood pressure.

      i. A narrow-complex tachycardia is generally supraventricular. **Adenosine** 0.05 to 0.2 mg/kg (up to 12 mg in adults) can be diagnostic as well as therapeutic because it temporarily blocks conduction through the AV node. This usually terminates a reentrant accessory pathway. An atrial tachycardia is generally "unmasked" during the period of AV block, allowing only p-waves to be seen on the ECG and therefore permitting easy calculation of the atrial rate. *Note:* Adenosine is an extremely short-acting drug, with a half-life of seconds. It must be given by rapid IV push followed immediately by a normal saline bolus, also by IV push. Although central access is preferable, it is not readily available. Peripheral IV access is an effective portal of drug entry as long as the medication is given rapidly.

      ii. A wide-complex tachycardia should be treated as ventricular tachycardia until proven otherwise. If the patient has a pulse, perform *synchronized cardioversion* 0.5 to 1 J/kg. After cardioversion, give **lidocaine** 1 mg/kg IV load. For a patient without a pulse, perform *asynchronous defibrillation* 2 to 4 J/kg.

REFERENCES

American Heart Association and American Association of Pediatrics: Cardiac rhythm disturbances. In *Textbook of pediatric life support*, 1994.

Chameides L: Dysrhythmias. In Barkin RM: *Pediatric emergency medicine*, ed 2, St Louis, 1997, Mosby.

D. Pulseless Electrical Activity (PEA)

RICHARD BACHUR

Electromechanical dissociation (EMD) is a form of PEA. Patients display signs of inadequate cardiac output and have no palpable pulses despite organized electrical activity on the ECG monitor.

Causes of Electromechanical Dissociation

1. Hypovolemia (volume loss, or relative hypovolemia in low–vascular tone states).
2. Tension pneumothorax.
3. Pericardial tamponade.
4. Cardiac or aortic rupture.
5. Pulmonary embolism.
6. Acidosis, hypoxemia.
7. Hypocalcemia.

Resuscitation

1. **Airway:** Secure the airway.
2. **Breathing:** Hyperventilate with 100% oxygen, intubate the trachea.

3. **Circulation:** Check for pulses and begin chest compressions.
   a. **Epinephrine** 0.01 mg/kg (0.1 ml/kg of 1:10,000) IV/IO, if given via ETT 0.1 mg/kg (10 times the usual dose except in newborns).
   b. Second and subsequent doses of epinephrine should be 10 times the initial dose, so-called high dose epi 0.1 mg/kg (0.1 ml/kg, 1:1000).
   c. Repeat every 3 minutes followed by a fluid flush.
   d. Monitor rhythm: EMD implies sinus rhythm with absence of pulses.
   e. Obtain access. After access is secured, routine laboratory tests for determining the cause of EMD include rapid glucose, ABG, electrolytes with calcium, and CBC (spun Hct). Obtain a type and crossmatch.
4. After initial assessment of the ABCs, control of airway and breathing, and initiation of chest compressions, begin a systematic approach to EMD based on the history and physical examination findings. If no single etiology is identified,
   a. Treat hypovolemia first with isotonic crystalloid 20 ml/kg.
   b. If no response occurs and still no specific etiology is obvious, empirically perform bilateral thoracentesis (for presumed tension pneumothorax) followed by bilateral chest tube placement. (See Thoracentesis [p. 12] in Chapter 2.)
   c. If no response to the above steps, consider pericardiocentesis.
   d. Continue to push volume, repeat isotonic crystalloid 20 ml/kg, and consider **O-negative blood,** especially with a history of trauma.
   e. Give **sodium bicarbonate** 1 mEq/kg if patient is acidotic.
   f. Recheck airway if patient is hypoxemic.

Diagnostic Aids

1. Hypovolemia: Should be considered first in all patients with EMD; obvious in instances of hemorrhage.
2. Tension pneumothorax: Shift of trachea, asymmetric breath sounds, distended neck veins, CXR finding.
3. Pericardial tamponade: Distant heart sounds, low-voltage ECG, distended neck veins. Pericardial tamponade should be strongly considered in patients with central venous lines.
4. Pulmonary embolism (PE): ECG changes (S-wave in lead I, Q-wave in lead III, T-wave in lead III, and right bundle branch block), loud S_2; PE should be considered in postoperative cardiac patients and those with indwelling central venous catheter, history of hypercoagulable states (including birth control pills, progesterone implants, systemic lupus erythematosus, nephrosis, severe dehydration, oncologic disease), atrial fibrillation, or prolonged immobilization.

REFERENCES

American Heart Association and American Association of Pediatrics: Cardiac rhythm disturbances. In *Textbook of pediatric life support*, 1994.

6. INITIAL APPROACH TO TRAUMA

MARK G. ROBACK

The trauma team typically comprises emergency department personnel, trauma surgeons, anesthesiologists, radiologists, and appropriate surgical specialty services, all with preassigned roles in providing emergency care to trauma victims.

History

Severe mechanisms and injuries with a high probability of serious injury include:
1. Mechanisms.
   a. Falls, typically more than two stories or 20 to 30 feet.
   b. Motor vehicle collisions.
      i. Extensive vehicular damage.
      ii. Roll-overs.
      iii. Ejection from vehicle.
      iv. Death of another vehicle occupant.
      v. Pedestrians struck by vehicles.
   c. Fires.
   d. Explosions.
   e. Sports injuries.
   f. Bicycle-related injuries.
2. Injuries.
   a. Penetrating trauma.
   b. Spinal cord injuries.
   c. Burns of the head or face that may lead to airway compromise, burns greater than 30% body surface area.
   d. More than two long bone fractures.
   e. Near or complete amputations proximal to the wrist or ankle.

Physical Examination

Primary survey: Identify and treat life-threatening conditions.
A **Airway**: Control with attention to control of the cervical spine.
B **Breathing**: Effort and effectiveness of ventilation.
C **Circulation**: With control of bleeding.
D **Disability**: Neurologic status.
E **Exposure**: The patient must be completely undressed.
   Environmental: Check core temperature, keep the patient warm.

Resuscitation

As the team progresses through the primary survey, any life-threatening process identified must have treatment initiated before the primary survey is continued.

1. Administer 100% oxygen, have suction available, control airway, maintain in-line alignment (head tilt contraindicated), perform rapid sequence intubation (RSI) if indicated. (See pp. 10 and 11 in Chapter 2 for detail on control of the cervical spine and RSI.)
2. Provide bag-valve-mask–assisted ventilation as indicated. Remember cricoid pressure to prevent aspiration of stomach contents in patients receiving positive-pressure ventilation.
3. IV access, two large-bore peripheral catheters, isotonic crystalloid 20 ml/kg as indicated. Repeat crystalloid bolus once, and then move to colloid and O-negative blood if type and crossmatched blood is not available.

Monitors

ECG and pulse oximeter, end-tidal CO_2 if intubated.

Radiology

In cases of major blunt trauma, three basic screening films are obtained—anteroposterior (AP) chest, AP pelvis, and lateral cervical spine.

Secondary Survey

A complete physical examination (head to toe) beginning with vital signs, including full examination of all body parts, and paying attention to areas not readily exposed (e.g., back, rectal examination).

Definitive Care

Initial stabilization by the trauma team is followed by definitive surgical care. May require transport to a trauma center.

REFERENCES

Committee on Trauma, American College of Surgeons: *Advanced trauma life support: course for physicians*, Chicago, 1993, American College of Surgeons, pp 17-37.

Fitzmaurice LS: Approach to multiple trauma. In Barkin RM: *Pediatric emergency medicine: concepts and clinical practice*, ed 2, St Louis, 1997, Mosby.

Ziegler MM, Templeton JM: Major trauma. In Fleisher GR, Ludwig S, eds: *Textbook of pediatric emergency medicine*, ed 3, Baltimore, 1993, Williams & Wilkins, pp 1089-1101.

7. INITIAL APPROACH TO NEONATAL RESUSCITATION

DEBRA WEINER

Delivery and resuscitation of the newborn should take place in the emergency department or clinic setting only when time does not permit transport to the delivery room.

The pregnant woman and neonate each require separate care providers (teams). Ideally, each team has a minimum of two health care professionals and at least one physician. Recognition that equipment requirements are different for delivery and newborn resuscitation is important. (See p. 4 in Chapter 1.)

Maternal History

1. Maternal age, gravida, para, aborta, prenatal care, estimated date of confinement based on last menstrual period or ultrasound, labor history (contractions, rupture of membranes, fetal movement, bleeding, trauma).
2. Pregnancy complications: Anemia, diabetes, preeclampsia, bleeding, infections, medications, tobacco, alcohol, drug use.
3. Previous pregnancy problems, previous cesarean section.

Maternal Physical Examination

1. ABCs.
2. Vital signs, including temperature.
3. Physical examination, including palpation of the abdomen to establish fetal position, fetal heart rate, and intensity and frequency of contractions.
4. Vaginal discharge for amniotic fluid (as determined using nitrazine paper), blood, and meconium.
5. *No speculum or digital examination of the vagina or rectum if bleeding is present.*

Potential Complications and Concerns

1. Delivery: Meconium, nuchal cord, shoulder dystocia, multiple gestation, postpartum hemorrhage, breech presentation, neonatal hypothermia.
2. Neonatal resuscitation: Respiratory depression, respiratory immaturity, meconium, pneumothorax, bradycardia, acidosis, hypovolemia, hypoglycemia, neonatal sepsis, fetal anomalies, neonatal depression as result of maternal narcotic, hypothermia.

Note: In neonatal resuscitation remember the importance of drying, stimulation, and maintaining the neonate's body temperature.

APGAR Score (Table 4-1)

1-Minute APGAR:

    7-10: Excellent; requires only drying, warming, stimulation, and suction.
    4-7: Moderately depressed; may require resuscitation.
    0-3: Severely depressed; immediate resuscitation required.

5-Minute APGAR: Aids in assessment of long-term outcome.

10-Minute APGAR: Should be performed if 5-minute APGAR <7.

Intubation

See Table 4-2.

Medications

See Table 4-3.

Table 4-1   *APGAR Score*

	Score		
	0	**1**	**2**
Heart rate	0	<100	>100
Respirations	None	Irregular, slow	Regular, crying
Muscle tone	None	Some flexion	Good flexion
Grimace	None	Requires stimulation	Spontaneous
Color	Pale or blue	Centrally pink,	Pink peripherally blue

Table 4-2   *Oral Airway Size and Endotracheal Tube Size for Neonatal Resuscitation*

Gestational Age (weeks)	Weight (g)	Oral Airway Size	ETT size (mm)
<28	<1000	000	2.5
28-34	1000-2000	000-00	3
34-38	2000-3000	00-0	3.5
>38	>3000	0	3.5-4.0

Table 4-3   *Medications Used in Neonatal Resuscitation*

Medication	Dose and Route	Indications
Epinephrine	0.1 to 0.3 ml/kg; 1:10,000 solution, IV, ETT	Bradycardia, asystole
Volume expander 5% Albumin Whole blood NS/RL	10 ml/kg IV over 5-10 min	Hypovolemia
Sodium bicarbonate	0.5-1 mEq/kg IV over >2 min	Metabolic acidosis
Naloxone	0.1 mg/kg IV, ETT, IM, SQ	Maternal narcotics
Dopamine	5 μg/kg/min initial; max 20 μg/kg/min continuous IV infusion	Persistent shock not responsive to volume

REFERENCES

American Heart Association and American Academy of Pediatrics: *Textbook of neonatal resuscitation*, 1988.

Berry LM, Padbury JF: Newborn resuscitation. In Barkin RM: *Pediatric emergency medicine: concepts and clinical practice*, ed 2, St Louis, 1997, Mosby.

Schafermeyer, RW: Neonatal resuscitation. In Fleisher GR, Ludwig S, eds: *Textbook of pediatric emergency medicine*, ed 3, Baltimore, 1993, Williams & Wilkins, pp 32-43.

8. INITIAL APPROACH TO INGESTIONS

ERICA LIEBELT

The initial approach to a child or adolescent with a known or suspected ingestion involves four basic phases: initial stabilization (life support), evaluation, detoxification, and supportive care.

Initial Stabilization (Life Support)

1. ABCs plus D (disability); level of consciousness, pupillary size.
2. Specific drugs may be needed to treat emergency side effects of many poisonings (Table 4-4).
3. Decontamination.
    a. Ocular: Saline lavage.
    b. Skin: Copious water.
    c. Gastrointestinal: Need for emergency GI decontamination must be based on history, potential for serious toxicity, and clinical presentation.

Table 4-4   Therapeutic Drugs for Side Effects of Poisoning

Ingestion or Exposure	Therapeutic Drugs
Carbon monoxide	Oxygen
Oral hypoglycemic agents, ethanol	Glucose
Narcotic overdose	Naloxone
Benzodiazepine overdose	Flumazenil
Tricyclic antidepressants (TCA)	Anticonvulsants
TCAs, cocaine, sympathomimetics	Antiarrhythmics

Evaluation

1. History—brief and focused.
    a. Identification of toxin.
    b. Route and time of exposure.
    c. Estimate of amount.
    d. Early symptoms.
    e. Home treatment.
    f. Suspect a toxic exposure if:
        i. Acute onset of symptoms.
        ii. Age <5 years.
        iii. History of pica or previous ingestions.
        iv. Household or environmental "stress."
        v. "Story does not make sense."
2. Physical examination.
    a. Clinical signs may be associated with specific drugs and chemicals (Table 4-5).
    b. Constellations of symptoms and signs produce a "toxidrome" typical of certain poisonings or classes of poisonings that will direct the therapeutic approach in a poisoning of unknown etiology.

Table 4-5   *Clinical Signs of Chemical Ingestion*

Clinical Sign	Ingestion
Coma	Barbiturates, benzodiazepines, carbon monoxide, cyanide, ethanol, opiates, TCAs
Fever	Anticholinergics, cocaine, salicylates, amphetamines
Hypothermia	Barbiturates, carbamazepine, ethanol, opiates
Hypertension	Amphetamines, cocaine, antihistamines
Hypotension	Beta-blockers, calcium channel blockers, barbiturates, benzodiazepines, clonidine, opiates
Tachypnea	Amphetamines, cocaine, salicylates, iron
Hypoventilation	Benzodiazepines, barbiturates, opiates
Breath odors	
Bitter almond	Cyanide
Garlic	Arsenic, organophosphates
Mothballs	Naphthalene, paradichlorobenzene
Fruit	Acetone, isopropanol
Miosis	Opiates, organophosphates, phenothiazines, clonidine
Mydriasis	Amphetamines, anticholinergics, cocaine

3. Laboratory tests (must be individualized).
   a. Quantitative serum drug levels (acetaminophen, salicylates, digoxin, carbon monoxide, theophylline, ethanol, anticonvulsants, and TCAs).
   b. Anion gap (difference between serum cations [Na^+] and anions [Cl^- and HCO_3^-]).
      i. Normal is approximately 12 mEq/L.
      ii. High anion gap metabolic acidosis (methanol, uremia, diabetic ketoacidosis, paraldehyde, isoniazid, iron, lactic acid, ethylene glycol, ethanol, salicylate, formaldehyde).
   c. Osmolality gap: Difference between measured and calculated osmoles.

$$2Na^+ + BUN/2.8 + glucose/18$$

   Can be explained by presence of methanol, ethylene glycol, ethanol, and isopropyl alcohol.
   d. Chest and abdominal radiographs (radiopacities, lead, foreign bodies).
   e. 12-Lead ECG.
   f. CBC, electrolytes, BUN/creatinine, glucose, ABG, serum osmolality, pregnancy test.
   g. Comprehensive toxicologic screen (rarely helpful in initial management because of turnaround time delay).

Detoxification

1. Reassess ABCs, and address compromises found.
2. GI decontamination—depending on specific toxin and clinical situation.
   a. Gastric lavage.
   b. Activated charcoal.
   c. Whole bowel irrigation.
3. Urgent antidotal therapy (Table 4-6).

Supportive Care

Table 4-6   *Urgent Antidotal Therapy*

Ingested Drug	Antidotal Therapy
Acetaminophen	*N*-Acetylcysteine (Mucomyst)
Digoxin	Digibind (Fab antibodies)
Iron	Deferoxamine
Cyanide	Sodium nitrite, sodium thiosulfate
Methemoglobinemic agents	Methylene blue
Organophosphates	Atropine, pralidoxime
Carbon monoxide	Oxygen
Isoniazid	Pyridoxine
Methanol, ethylene	Ethanol

Continued monitoring of:

1. ABCs.
2. Fluid and electrolyte status.
3. Level of consciousness.

REFERENCES

Pratt J: Signs and symptoms of acute disorders in children—coma. In May HL, Aghababian RV, Fleisher GR, eds: *Emergency medicine*, ed 2, Boston, 1992, Little, Brown, p 1792.

Tennenbein M: General management principles of poisoning. In Barkin RM: *Pediatric emergency medicine: concepts and clinical practice*, ed 2, St Louis, 1997, Mosby.

A Mock Code Checklist

_____ Code leader identified, roles designated   _____

_____ Gloves, masks, eye protection   _____

_____ Estimated weight in kg = $(2 \times$ Age in yr $+ 9)$ _____

Primary Survey—ABCs

Airway   _____ Neutral neck position, do not hyperextend, jaw thrust/chin lift,   _____
C-spine?

Breathing   _____ Effective respirations, chest movement   _____

   _____ Obstruction? Suction   _____

   _____ Bag-mask with 100% O_2 _____

   _____ Intubation: O_2, medications, ETT size, stylet, laryngoscope,   _____
position, tape, NG tube

Circulation   _____ Assessment, carotid vs. brachial/femoral, perfusion, color/mottling   _____

   _____ Compressions: position, counting, backboard   _____

   _____ IV access, appropriate fluid resuscitation   _____

   _____ Resuscitation medications   _____

Disability   _____ Brief neurologic assessment (GCS, pupils)   _____

Exposure   _____ Remove obstructing clothing   _____

Secondary Survey

_____ History

_____ Physical examination: complete (rectal, back)

_____ Monitors (ECG/oximeter/capnometer)

_____ Rapid glucose by fingerstick

_____ Hematocrit

_____ Temperature

_____ ABG/laboratory tests

_____ Reassess—continuous

Additional

_____ Assessment of fluids given

_____ Additional medications (e.g., pressors)

_____ Cardioversion/defibrillation

_____ Tubes: Foley, NG/OG, chest tube

_____ Radiology department called for appropriate studies

_____ Surgical consults if indicated

_____ Appropriate interaction with parents/family

           End Time   _____

COMMENTS:

B Mock Code Scenario Template

[AUTHOR]

Objectives

1.
2.
3.

Brief Presenting History

Initial Vital Signs

If asked: T   °C (R)
Estimated weight: kg

Initial Physical Examination

General appearance:
If asked:
- **Airway:**
- **Breathing:**
- **Circulation:**

Further History Given on Request

Expected interventions	Complications
1.	
2.	
3.	
4.	
5.	

Repeat Vital Signs

Progression

Laboratory Tests

Options

Expected interventions	Complications
1.	
2.	
3.	
4.	
5.	

Additional Potential Complications

Disposition

Discussion of Objectives

Additional Comments

REFERENCES

C Pediatric Approximate Size and Normal Values Chart

Age	Wt (kg)	RR (rpm)	HR (bpm)	BP systolic (mm Hg)	Suction catheter (Fr)
Premie	<3	<60	140	52 ± 10	6
Newborn	3-4	<60	125	60 ± 10	8
1-6 mo	4-6	24-30	140	80 ± 10	10
6-12 mo	6-10		135	89 ± 25	10
1-2 yr	10-13	20-24	120	96 ± 30	10
2-4 yr	13-17		110	99 ± 25	10-14
4-6 yr	17-20		100	100 ± 20	14
6-8 yr	20-25	12-20	100	105 ± 13	14-16
8-10 yr	25-30		90	110 ± 15	16
10-12 yr	30-40		80	112 ± 15	16
12-14 yr	40-50		80	115 ± 20	16
14-adult	>50	10-14	70	120 ± 20	16

Laryngoscope	ETT (mm)	Trach size (Fr)	NG (Fr)	Foley	Chest tube (Fr)
0 Miller	2.5-3.0	00	5	5	10
0 Miller	3.0-3.5	0	8	5	10-12
1 Miller	3.5-4.0	0-1	8	8	10-12
1 Miller	4.0	1-2	8	8	12-20
1 Miller	4.5	1-2	8	8-10	16-20
1-2 Miller	5.0	2-3	8-10	10	20-24
2 Miller	5.5 + cuffed	3	10	10	24-28
2 Miller	6.0 cuffed	3-4	10	10	28
2 Miller	6.0-7.0 cuffed	4	10-12	10-12	28-32
2 Miller 2 Mac	7.0 cuffed	4-5	12	12	32
2-3 Miller 2-3 Mac	7.0-7.5 cuffed	5-6	12	12	32-36
3 Miller 3 Mac	7.5-8.0 cuffed	6	14	12	36-42

D Abbreviations

ABCs	airway, breathing, and circulation	**DOCA**	deoxycortisone acetate
ABG	arterial blood gas	**DPL**	diagnostic peritoneal lavage
ACTH	adrenocorticotropic hormone	**ECG or**	
AF	anterior fontanel	**EKG**	electrocardiogram
ALT	alanine aminotransferase	**EEG**	electroencephalogram
AMS	acute mountain sickness	**EMD**	electromechanical dissociation
AP	anteroposterior	**EMT**	emergency medical technician
ARDS	acute respiratory distress syndrome, adult respiratory defense syndrome	**ENT**	ear, nose, and throat surgeons
		ETT	endotracheal tube
ASAP	as soon as possible	**FB**	foreign body
AST	aspartate aminotransferase	**FFP**	fresh frozen plasma
AV	atrioventricular	**Fr**	French
AVM	arterial-venous malformation	**GCS**	Glasgow Coma Scale
ax	axial	**GI**	gastrointestinal
BAT	blunt abdominal trauma	**GTC**	generalized tonic-clonic
BP	blood pressure	**GU**	genitourinary
BPM	beats per minute	**HACE**	high-altitude cerebral edema
BUN	blood urea nitrogen	**HAPE**	high-altitude pulmonary edema
BVM	bag-valve-mask	**Hct**	hematocrit
CAH	congenital adrenal hyperplasia	**HEENT**	head, eyes, ears, nose, and throat
CBC	complete blood count (usually includes differential and platelets)	**Hgb**	hemoglobin
		HR	heart rate
CHF	congestive heart failure	**HUS**	hemolytic-uremic syndrome
CNS	central nervous system	**ICP**	intracranial pressure
CO	carbon monoxide	**ICU**	intensive care unit
CPP	cerebral perfusion pressure	**IM**	intramuscular
CPR	cardiopulmonary resuscitation	**IO**	intraosseous
Cr	creatinine	**ITP**	idiopathic (immune) thrombocytopenia
CR	cardiorespiratory	**IUGR**	intrauterine growth retardation
CSF	cerebrospinal fluid	**IV**	intravenous
C-spine	cervical spine	**IVF**	intravenous fluid
CT	computed tomography	**IVP**	intravenous push
CVA	cerebral-vascular accident (stroke)	**JVD**	jugular venous distention
CVL	central venous line	**LFT**	liver function test
CVP	central venous pressure	**LOC**	loss of consciousness
CXR	chest x-ray	**LRI**	lower respiratory infection
DIC	disseminated intravascular coagulation	**LUQ**	left upper quadrant
DKA	diabetic ketoacidosis	**Mac**	MacIntosh blade

MAP	mean arterial pressure		**rpm**	respirations per minute
MAST	military antishock trousers		**RR**	respiratory rate
MCD	mock code director		**RSI**	rapid sequence intubation
MRI	magnetic resonance imaging		**RSV**	respiratory syncytial virus
NC	nasal cannula		**RVH**	right ventricular hypertrophy
NG	nasogastric [tube]		**SE**	status epilepticus
NICU	newborn intensive care unit		**SIADH**	syndrome of inappropriate secretion of antidiuretic hormone
NKDA	no known drug allergies			
NS	normal saline		**SIDS**	sudden infant death syndrome
NSVD	normal, spontaneous, vaginal delivery		**SL**	sublingual
OG	orogastric		**SLE**	systemic lupus erythematosus
OR	operating room		**SQ**	subcutaneous
ORL	otolaryngologist (ENT surgeon)		**SVR**	systemic vascular resistance
P	pulse		**SVT**	supraventricular tachycardia
PDA	patent ductus arteriosus		**T**	temperature
PE	phenytoin equivalent		**TCA**	tricyclic antidepressant
PEA	pulseless electrical activity		**TIBC**	total iron-binding capacity
PEEP	positive end expiratory pressure		**type and**	
PERRL	pupils equal, round, and reactive to light		**cross**	type and crossmatch blood
			UA	urinalysis
PICU	pediatric intensive care unit		**UAC**	umbilical artery catheter
PIP	peak inspiratory pressure		**UC**	urine culture
PIV	peripheral IV		**URI**	upper respiratory infection
Plts	platelets		**UVC**	umbilical vein catheterization
PO	per os (mouth)		**VBG**	venous blood gas
PR	per rectum		**VF or**	
PRCBs	packed red blood cells		**V-fib**	ventricular fibrillation
PRN	as needed		**VP**	ventriculoperitoneal
PT	prothrombin time		**VSD**	ventricular septal defect
PTT	partial thromboplastin time		**VT or**	
RA	room air		**V-tach**	ventricular tachycardia
RAD	reactive airways disease		**WBC**	white blood cell count
RL	Ringer's lactate solution			

E ECG Rhythms

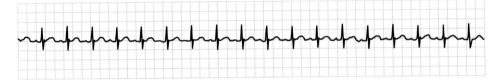

Normal sinus rhythm—110 bpm

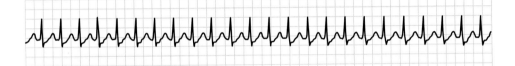

Normal sinus rhythm—144 bpm

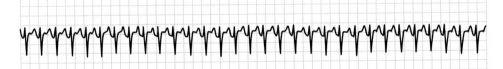

Sinus tachycardia—182 bpm

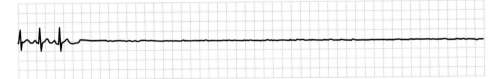

Asystole

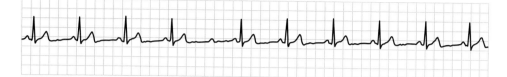

Bradycardia—60 bpm

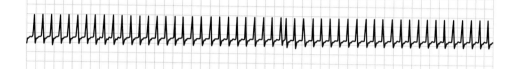

Supraventricular tachycardia—300 bpm

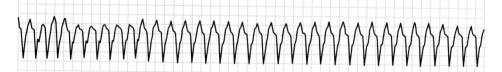

Ventricular tachycardia

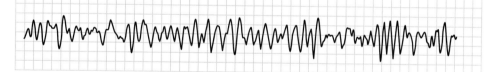

Ventricular fibrillation

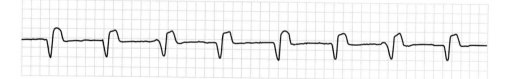

Idioventricular

F Glasgow Coma Scales

Behavior/Response	Score	Behavior/Response	Score
Adults		**Modified for Infants**	
Eye opening		*Eye opening*	
Spontaneously	4	Spontaneously	4
To speech	3	To speech	3
To pain	2	To pain	2
None	1	None	1
Best verbal response		*Verbal*	
Oriented	5	Coos, babbles	5
Confused	4	Irritable, cries	4
Inappropriate	3	Cries to pain	3
Incomprehensible	2	Moans to pain	2
None	1	None	1
Best motor response		*Motor*	
Obey commands	6	Normal spontaneous movements	6
Localize pain	5	Withdraws to touch	5
Withdrawal	4	Withdraws to pain	4
Flexion to pain	3	Abnormal flexion	3
Extension	2	None	1
None	1		

Index